Memoirs of a Machine:

The Book on Optimum Performance Nutrition For the Human Machine

By

John MACHINE Lober

If the Bible is (B)basic (I)instructions (B)before (L)leaving (E)Earth for the mind and soul, then John Lober's book on Optimum Performance Nutrition (OPN) is the instruction manual for the human body.

This book is dedicated to my Mom.

Published by Born to Fight Books
All rights reserved
Copyright ©2014
John Lober

Introduction

As a Mixed-Martial Artist your body is like a Machine. The Machine doesn't run on exercise. It runs on the food you put in your mouth. When you place the proper food or fuel in your Machine and you train at high level, the level of achievement becomes infinite. e, hence, the Optimum Performance Level (OPL) for a Human Machine. What I am about to explain to you is just so totally practical, you will have trouble comprehending that it actually works, so, It's time to feed the Machine properly.

My name is John MACHINE Lober. I am the creator and prime operator of Machine Martial Arts Worldwide and Machine Fit personal training since 1995. I was a world class mixed martial arts champion in the late 90's, with a notable win over the Legendary Frank Shamrock. I am an authority in mixed martial arts in all aspects, a trainer of champion athletes in many professional and amateur sports, Minister, and author of Memoirs of a Machine: Inside the Mind of a Cage fighter. I have not laid my sword to rest. I have changed battlefields to the battlefield of Wellness and Longevity in the quest for the ultimate in Optimum Performance Nutrition for the Human Machine.

Over four decades of my life, through trial and error, I have encountered and endured every physical type of training and diet that a blue-collar athlete can do. I wasn't an Olympic athlete and I wasn't a collegiate division one athlete and I didn't have a lot of the scholars directing me during my training, so I had to discover most of my research on my own. A majority of my younger years were spent in the Library reading volumes of books and always keeping up on the up and coming and new training methods, and how to manipulate my body through diet. My interests were the manipulation of the Hormonal system, increasing mass, losing weight and creating Optimum Performance in the athlete. This book is a conglomeration of all the good things that worked for me. Everybody's body is different, so some of the things that worked for me might not work for you. But, in general, the concept is the same for everyone. You can take the book of Optimum Performance Nutrition (OPN) for mixed martial arts and apply it to your own life and keep what works for you, discard the shit that doesn't. There is a fine line between proper nutrition and solid training that every serious athlete and fighter should understand. The goal of this book is to help you understand how to eat, why you eat and what you should eat to obtain Optimum Performance (OP) in any sport that you choose, but specifically Mixed Martial Arts. Also, the importance of cycling and periodization, what the difference is between training and just working out, and some obstacles and limitations I encountered, that I will help you avoid on your journey to becoming an efficient fighting Machine or just the best at whatever you choose. Stay strong and I hope you enjoy my no holds barred, brutally honest Memoir of my journey to obtain Optimum Performance Level (OPL) of the Machine.

TABLE OF CONTENTS

1. Prime Objective
2. Fuel
3. Training vs. Working Out
4. Running on Empty
5. Shutting Down
6. A Daily Journal
7. Supplements
8. Testimonials

Prologue

"You want some Nubain, Lobes?" Todd asked.

"Nah, Dude. I might like it too much and you know what that means." I replied.

After about a year of that carrot dangling in my face, I broke down. I was up to a lot mischief at this point in my life, so why not? I took it home and slammed it, reluctantly, but I did it. The room closed in on me. Squeezing my head to the point my vision was a pinhole, like looking out of a tunnel. My head was being squeezed in a vise. An elephant was standing on my skull or like I was a thousand feet deep in the ocean. Like being choked out. I braced myself, then quickly regained consciousness. I had no idea how much to use, now I do. I hurried to the gym to get a workout in and found it had a thirty-minute shelf life and I couldn't feel any pain. That's how you take it to the next level. I grew and grew and became stronger. The pain barrier was not an issue any longer.

1.   Prime Objective

You are an experienced trained athlete with martial arts training and you want to compete for the very first time? So, your metabolism has come to a screeching halt and your 50lbs over weight. Oh, you have a pencil neck and your ribs stick out and you want to beef up so you are not bullied anymore? You just had your second child and you have no idea how to lose this extra 40lbs? You are a full time mom, always eating the kids leftovers at McDonalds, you workout everyday and can't figure out why you're not losing?

When I was in High School my focus was always to gain weight. I was 175lbs my senior year and the coaches were always trying things to bulk me up. They moved me from Linebacker to Offensive center and the other four guys were 250 plus. I was drinking protein powder, milk and raw egg shakes every day. I even tried pounding a case of Ensure at one point in the quest for size. My coach was pumping my scrawny ass full of desiccated Liver tablets on a daily bases at one point. I was so bloated and irritable that I went to snap the ball and shit my pants on the field. A Hershey squirt. I went running back to the team room with a hash mark in the crack of my white practice pants. I graduated All-CIF Sunset League Center.

After High School, I was, for some reason, into lifting heavy weight, I think mainly to get big and strong to battle Bullies. So, my Dad got me a membership to Racquetball World behind the house. They couldn't get me to go home. There were a bunch of old timers there and they showed me my foundation for lifting. Legendary professional baseball players, NFL football guys, some cops, an ex football coach and firemen.

I remember a trip to the 1985 Olympics in LA to watch Olympic Powerlifting. I heard of places like the Olympic training center in Colorado, and places like the Nebraska Cornhuskers Training center. I never actually made it to these places, they were just places I heard of. I did my best, every time I worked out, to visualize myself actually being there and what it must have been like.

My best friend and I had an idea to go to Tijuana and get this stuff I read about in the library called Dianabol, D Bol, from West Germany. Little blue tablets in a foil press pack. 80/ 2 mg pack of pills for $20. Oh man, that shit worked. And it was an Anabolic. The only side effect of that shit was size and strength, but they soon discontinued manufacturing it, and that was over soon enough. FYI, for all you guys that think steroids are still badass, I bet you didn't know that they aren't even as effective as they should be unless your taking a thyroid. But hey, good luck with that.

After that cycle, I began to focus on cardiovascular endurance to be a Fireman. Those silly aerobic classes that were a fad in the 80's. They made me do it in the Academy. I went into running and sprinting at the local College after that, which became a regular staple in my life to this day. But I was always focusing on gaining weight. My mother would always scream at me for eating all the groceries. I slept 12 to 16 hours at a time and I would eat all night long. A box of Rice Crispies in a salad bowl with half a gallon of milk with artificial sweetener sprinkled on top. Or, a pound of cooked spaghetti with a jar of Marinara sauce with a block of sharp cheddar cheese. I could eat three charbroiled chicken sandwiches on the way home from Thanksgiving dinner at my girlfriend's house, no problem. I ate and I lifted.

2. Fuel
It's a diet lifestyle. I am going to tell you something that is going to change your life forever. This is a concept so practical that you wont believe it at first. Dieting is a state of mind and a change of lifestyle. A proper diet will give you an endless supply of energy and a physique you will be proud of. Diet meaning eating. My diet tolerates zero outside influence from recreational drugs and or prescription drugs. No alcoholic beverages or carbonated beverages like soda. The carbonation neutralizes the stomach acid and inhibited the absorption of nutrients from your food that you eat. No simple sugars, (see carbohydrates) or margarines. Butter is all right but not for weight loss. Replace that with fish oils and olive oil for cooking. Discontinue all processed foods, they have little or no nutritional value whatsoever and can create other health problems not yet discovered by the FDA and also, eating un-nutritional foods leads to illness like the flu. And, also discontinue as much bread as you can. White bread is actually better than the whole-wheat stuff because it takes longer to digest. Also, I like to eat foods that are high in fiber, mainly greens like broccoli, green beans and kale. These increase the metabolism during digestion and give the intestine something to squeeze on to keep your metabolism burning hot. I don't have a problem with having a cup of coffee or tea, just don't over do it. Definitely do not use any artificial sweeteners. This shit gives me lead feet and I read that it converts to formaldehyde. If you just follow those few rules or restrictions, and dismiss that stuff from your diet, you see a drastic change in your energy level in as little as four weeks or less. It's a huge difference in most people's lives because pretty much our society is operating below a baseline, a rock bottom level. Therefore, any thing you do, you will notice the significance of the change

for the better.

Sadness. Worry. Doubt. Confusion. Anger. Depression. Rage. Underlying feelings.

That was what I was really fighting. It was a huge, ugly, fuckin' monster. Talk about fear; I feared it to death. Beneath the anger was fear. The Angst. I had fear of gassing out in a fight, fear of the unknown, and fear of not measuring up. I had sadness and depression of dead relatives and friends. Or from being bullied. Men and women have their reasons for bad feelings and this is what's making them fat. Food was giving me hope, was giving me good feelings, which I used to balance my bad feelings. But then, the balance was off. I needed to find a way to deal with it.

Food is a Drug. Psychologically, that sort of thing is spoken of a lot today, especially in regard to people who have a lot of pain in their lives. We would say they medicate their pain with food. They anesthetize themselves to the hurt inside by eating, but this isn't some rare, technical syndrome. All of us do it. Everybody. No exceptions.

We all ease our discomfort using food and cover our unhappiness by setting our eyes on dinnertime. Fasting exposes all of us: our pain, our pride, our anger. Fast for twenty-four hours and your true character will be revealed. Either you will fight or submit. If anger controls us, it will be revealed almost immediately.

MACHINE FIT
PRIVATE PERSONAL TRAINING
with John Lober

Food is a drug. It's the number one drug that is

abused by everyone on this planet. It makes us feel good. Just try to fast for 24 hours and you will see what exactly you are made of. You will either fight, or you will roll over and submit. Remember, any trainer that offers you a prescription or street drug, as a shortcut to obtaining your fitness and wellness goals is a FOOL.

THE BASIC DIET FACTS

Water is an essential nutrient even though it is left out of discussions pertaining to your body's nutritional needs. Your body's need for water is second only to that of oxygen. Water is used by the body as a building material, lubricant, solvent, and helps regulate your body temperature. It is used by the body as a solvent and after digestion, water and blood are the means by which nutrients are carried to your cells and wastes are removed. Remember, people stranded or lost in the wild can only survive 48-72 hours without water. You can go without food for up to 20-30 days! Water is vital to not only survival, but, optimal health and performance!

How much should I drink?
For people who are used to drinking a lot of water should first start out with drinking a half to one gallon a day. It sounds like a lot but if you keep on sipping all-day it will be gone in no time.
When the weather is hot and humid, make a conscious effort to increase fluid intake. Don't wait until you are thirsty, if you rely on thirst you will only be replacing 50-70/% of the fluid you have lost. A good self-monitoring method of your state of hydration is to look at your urine. A dark gold color means you are dehydrated. A pale yellow or clear color means you are headed toward a state of hydration. You might want to limit or even stay clear of caffeine and alcohol because they can act like

diuretics, dehydrating you.

1. PROTEIN

Don't forget the eggs, chicken, dairy, lean beef, and fish. Bottom line: Mix it up! Remember, unless you're a big bag of laziness, in which case you won't last very long in this game anyway, you'll be eating five or more meals per day every two or three hours. Over those five meals you need to divide your protein intake (not necessarily equally) and eat protein from a variety of sources. It's all about balance.

I love steak. When I eat steak it converts into steroids in my stomach and bulks me up. If I eat fish or chicken only, I get too lean and I lose muscle mass. If I eat all three and mix it up every meal, I find that happy medium.

2. FAT

The best sources for any dietary fats are organic plants and animals. These are plants that are gown in healthy soil according to the principles of traditional farming, without any chemical sprays, pesticides, fungicides and so on. Organic animals are raised in a healthy, natural environment where they can move around, fed the diet they would eat in nature, and not subjected to hormones, steroids or unnecessary antibiotics. The problem is that most people nowadays, trying to "save money" on food, do not eat these types of foods, but rather consume pesticide-sprayed, genetically-modified vegetables and commercially-raised animals that have been poisoned with cheap and incorrect foods, living in inhumane living conditions. And about 100% of commercially farmed animals are on drugs. Since the body stores toxins in fat, when commercially-raised animals are fed interesting items such as cardboard, newspaper, wood chips, cement dust and manure - all approved by the FDA for animal feed - the liver cannot handle the toxic overload and pushes the excess into fat. This causes the huge weight gain - up to 30% - in cattle fed cement dust. This is great for the farmer who gets paid for his animals by the pound, but not so good for the animal itself, or for you! Prime cuts of meat are generally marbled with fat, so if the animal is not organically raised and grass-fed, you are eating the animal's toxin stores along with your filet mignon. So, eat a variety of healthy fats from various organic meats, eggs, avocados, olives, nuts, seeds, coconut, flax seeds, and other recommended oils. Don't be scared about these, they are extremely beneficial and vital for our overall health!

3. CARBOHYDRATES

First of all, keep in mind that approximately 75% of the American population simply does not do well with carbs. As such, try to eat carbohydrate foods that score below 50 on the glycemic indexThe obvious exception to this is post workout, when it is recommended that you do eat high GI carbs, along with protein. Secondly, simply eat more vegetables-a lot more vegetables. That simple trick alone will help you burn fat. You might also consider gorging on the cruciferous vegetables like broccoli, cauliflower, and cabbage.

Here's an example:

When we eat carbohydrates, they are digested, and then turn into blood sugar. Our body asks do we need this sugar? (For energy stores in our muscles or for other reactions in our bodies) If we've just worked out and our energy stores are low, then our bodies use the sugar and shuttle onto our muscles to restore energy levels. If we aren't active, then our bodies say NO, we don't need it, store it away. This is when our body stores excess sugars and grains away as fat stores...remember, we are not fat from eating too much fat...the majority of our problem comes from eating way too many grains, sugars and processed foods.

There are two types of carbohydrates, simple and complex. Simple carbs are sugars that are broken down quickly by the body for energy. Table sugar, Honey, Fruit and Jelly are some examples of Simple carbs. Complex carbs are rich in fiber and high in vitamins and minerals. Green vegetables, Whole grains, and Beans are examples of complex carbs.

4. MICRONUTRIENTS (Vitamins and Minerals)
Nutrients from food are absorbed by the body as it passes through the digestive system: Nutrients are essential for cell growth, maintenance and repair. Nutrients provide energy to enable your body to function efficiently. Nutrients, along with fiber and water, are essential to your body to function efficiently. Nutrients, along with fiber and water, are essential to your good health. Although nutrients can work alone, each depends upon the others to be the most effective. The main nutrients are the macronutrients, carbohydrates, proteins, and fats - and the micronutrients, vitamins and minerals. For instance, try 3 cups of green vegetables, mainly Kale, because it is the densest in nutrients and the best way to replace and supplement nutrients and feed the Mitochondria in your cells. There is evidence that this can actually cure you of many diseases. Juicing is a great and efficient way to ingest these, as opposed to blending, which leaves in the fiber to work your digestive system just a little bit more and creating a fire to burn calories.

A. VITAMINS/ MINERALS

Vitamins and minerals do not in themselves provide energy, but macronutrients depend on them to regulate the release of energy from food. Vitamins are organic substances. They activate enzymes, which are proteins that act as catalysts to speed up biological reactions that take place in your body. Your body produces a certain amount of vitamins D and K, but all other vitamins come from your diet or supplementation.

B. OMEGA FATTY ACIDS

The evidence continues to roll in about all the good things fish oil can do for your health. Omega-3 fats are high in two fats that are crucial to your health – DHA and EPA. Scientific research indicates hat these compounds may help prevent a variety of very serious diseases including heart disease, cancer, diabetes, depression and more. Now it looks like a daily dose of fish oil, coupled with a moderate exercise plan, helps you lose weight too.

C. Importance of WHOLE FOODS

The core of good eating starts with eating whole foods: the real thing, grown in the ground, caught on the hook, raised on the range or laid in the nest. The difficult part is how to actually find the whole foods in America today.

Current statistics say that the FDA lists approximately 2800 international food additives and about 3,000 chemicals, which are deliberately added to our food supply. When considering the number of chemicals used in the process of growing and processing food, by the food to the time it reaches our stomach we have consumed between 10,000 and 15,000 chemicals a day!

The fact is, the average American eats approximately his or her body weight in food additives each year, or approximately 150 pounds; this statistic is roughly the same for most English speaking countries. Of this amount, 15 pounds or more will be used as flavoring agents, preservatives and dyes, many of which are considered GRAS by the FDA.

So, why all this talk about foods and stuff?
The number one weight loss stumbling block, a liver

overloaded with pollutants and toxins, cannot burn body fat, and thus will sabotage your weight/ fat loss efforts. You should also keep in mind that excessive toxins form conventional plant and animal foods overload your liver and encourage extra fat to form around your midsection, whether you are a man or a woman. The more toxic and/ or dehydrated you are. the thicker the layer of fluid becomes, making you appear chubbier or bloated. By eating organic, grass fed and free range food, you will see significant improvements in the results or your program. Do not overlook this advice!! It is a vital component of this program. Remember, food manufacturers are NOT required to prove that their products sustain life, Pretty much every research dollar they spend is to determine how to make foods cheaper, increase shelf life and how to trick you into buying them. Good healthy food requires little marketing because people know it's good for them from their own experience. They need to convince you to eat their garbage, so they need to spend a lot of marketing money to ensure you do. The longer it lasts on the shelf, the worse it is for you. Most things in nature will not last more than a few days once picked or killed for consumption. Increasing a product's shelf life means stripping it of anything that will eventually cause it to spoil, such as enzymes, vitamins, minerals and ultimately its life force. Many of the foods you eat today are so full of chemicals and pesticide residues you can leave them sitting on the kitchen counter for days on end and the ants won't even touch them - proving that the bugs are smarter than we are in regards to eating. Almost everything that comes fresh ahs been altered, whether its pesticides, hormones, growth stimulators, antibiotics, plastic hay (to add fiber to cattle diets), cooking oils tested with dry-cleaning chemicals, fish raised on dog chow…the list goes on.

This messing with the food supply began in the 1970's, when the FDA allowed congressional approval. Today, more than 70% of our food is genetically altered and we won't really know the consequences for decades.

The best place to find whole foods are at local markets and/ or organic local market (Whole Foods, Trader Joes, Mother's Market, Sprouts, etc...) BUT, beware, just because it's in these markets, doesn't mean it's safe and healthy. Be selective and make sure that the foods are organic and free of nasty pollutants and additives.

OK, so how much should I eat?

How to eat for ULTIMATE HEALTH and OPTIMUM PERFORMANCE LEVELS.

Congratulations on getting started!!

"The starting point of all achievement is desire. Keep this constantly in mind. Weak desires bring weak results, just as a small fire makes a small amount of heat."
Napoleon Hill
1883-1970, Author of Think and Grow Rich

"The 4 D's of success. Desire, Dedication, Discipline and Determination."-JL

The #1 key to ultimate health and an energetic life is healthy eating and optimum nutrition! Here are a few guidelines and tips...

Optimum performance was my goal, and this was essential to achieve it. I gained muscle and lost more body fat. I could train harder and longer and eat a lot more. I was probably burning up to 4,000 calories a day, eating 4,100 and burning all of my body fat off.

The concept was like a fireplace burning wood. Your metabolism is the fire. Three logs on the fire burn hot. When the fire is going out—about every three hours—you stoke it again with three more logs. It has to be three to get it to last another three hours and keep burning hot. If you put just a handful of twigs, it burns real hot and fast, and then goes out quickly. If you put five logs on, it smothers it. It smokes and chokes the fire out. This was the basic concept to increasing metabolism, and it worked.

Portion sizes and timing were important as well as the Glycemic Index. What's this? Well, it's the rate at which the carbs digest into your body, essentially. Some are good carbs and others are not as good. All carbohydrates are given a number from 1 to 100 based on their rate of absorption into the body. This is done for Diabetics so they can monitor the insulin levels in their body. Insulin is the key to nutrients entering the cells. It is desirable to not spike Insulin for weight loss and healthy living. If you hold a handful of steamed rice under hot water and squeeze, what happens? It liquefies. It does that inside you, too, rushing into your blood stream to give you a sugar rush. The body produces insulin to get it into the system, but then it crashes once that's done.

However, if you chop up some green apples and hold them under hot water and squeeze, what happens? Not much, actually. They take longer for the body to break down and therefore your metabolism has to work harder to digest this food. Now, to additionally slow this rate down, add a little peanut butter, or fat. I was getting good at the diet thing. Adding fat to every meal was like smearing hot wax over a screen on my stomach lining, allowing the food I digested to trickle into the blood stream with out the rush I was used to. And the fiber was giving my guts something to grab on to. My intestines were getting a workout from squeezing and twisting my food up while it breaks it down. That's what Metabolism is. Its hot from the constant workout it gets from the constant flow of food I was giving it.

Habit #1: Eat every 2-3 hours (6-8 meals per day)
This will require some preparation and planning on your part. Use alarms or reminders to help develop this habit. Use Tupperware and after a couple weeks, it will become routine and you can phase out of using these reminders.
Think of your metabolism as a fireplace. You want to keep it burning hot. They way you do that is you throw wood on it, or stoke the fireplace. You wouldn't throw ten logs on the fire because it would smother and snuff it out. You would just toss a handful of twigs on it because it wouldn't burn very long. So, the size or amount of wood or food your putting on your fire is very important. And the trick is to keep the metabolism or fire burning 24 hours a day.

Habit #2: Eat complete, healthy fats, veggies and/or fruits with every meal.
The simple fact is, our bodies work better with a balance of carbohydrates, fats and protein. Not only is protein essential for building healthy muscle and maintaining a strong immune system, it stabilizes insulin levels, which leads to steady energy throughout the day. One more benefit: eating protein has been shown to reduce your appetite. When possible, strive to eat organic foods that are free of hormones, pesticides, additives and other artificial ingredients.

The portion sizes of my meals are as important as scheduling. I don't measure. I judge the size of the meal and keep it the size of my fist, no larger. If you're 40 lbs over weight, and it takes your body 2 1/2 hours to digest the meal, it will search out other calories from with in your body and burn the fat for that extra thirty minutes. Any longer, will slow the metabolism down. A good rule of thumb is, if you think your meal is too large don't finish it all. Leave some on the plate.

To determine exact serving/ portion size, listen to your body approximately 30 minutes after you eat.
If you are hungry, you didn't eat enough
If you are sleepy, you ate too much.
If you feel great, you consumed just the right serving/ portion size.

Habit #3: Control portion sizes - The hand method is used to ensure you're eating healthy portions relative to your body size. Since you base your meal size on the size of your hand, men will likely be eating larger portions than women. While this method is an approximation, it will help keep your potion sizes reasonable. The hand method also serves as a good gauge when you are eating out. When in doubt, just don't finish everything on your plate and grazing is a good way to calorie restrict.
- Eat a salad or variety of veggies the size of both hands put together.
- Eat meats and poultry the size and thickness of the palm of your hand.
- Eat a handful of nuts or seeds per day.

Habit #4: Drink water all day! 75% of Americans are chronically dehydrated. One glass of water will shut down midnight hunger pangs for almost 100% of the dieters studied in a University of Washington study. Lack of water is the #1 trigger of daytime fatigue. Preliminary research indicates that 8-10 glasses of water a day could significantly ease back and joint pain for up to 80% of sufferers.

Hydration is important to keep the pipes flowing. Your digestive track and your cardiovascular system are in essence a tube inside of a tube. Hydration enables the process of waste removal and to carry nutrients to the cells. I drink about 8-10 cups of water a day. Sometimes I give it a splash of Apple Juice. I always have it ready to go in my fridge. One of the best tricks I know for jump-starting my metabolism is to drink cold water right when I wake up. I can feel it work as it goes down. If you don't drink water regularly, you can retain it or become dehydrated. I think of it as flushing the toilet.

Habit #5: Eat whole foods for most meals (except workout and immediate post-workout drinks) unless impossible, then use supplements (shakes and bars) when necessary.

Habit #6: Plan meal ahead of time.
You may even want to try different recipes and decide what works for you before you begin your training program. What works for me may be different from what foods work well for you. Along with food sensitivities and allergies, this is trial and error for you. Experiment with different seasonings, try a variety of vegetables, and find which microwave settings work best for preheating food, By the time you're ready to start, you'll have the supplies you need and the confidence that you know what you're doing. Then, fix your meals in advance and freeze them. It's important to shop at least once a week. If you forget, you'll run out of good food and be tempted to cheat on your diet.

Habit #7: Get containers to store your food.
Purchase plastic storage containers, sports bottles, a water jug and a cooler to store and carry your food. Having nutritious meals within reach during a hectic day can keep you on track and in the game. DON'T GET CAUGHT WITHOUT FOOD!

Habit #8: Strive for consistency, not perfection.
You can be sure there WILL be the occasional meal or snack that's not on the recommended food list. When you get off track in this way, don't allow it to slow you down. Enjoy the divergence, recommit to your goal, and get back on track with your very next meal.

Habit #9: FAST FOOD is poison.
I mean this stuff is cheaper than dog food, so you got to ask yourself why? But, what if I am stuck in the middle of nowhere and Arby's is all there is. Well, that's not going to kill you, but I bet you there is a grocery store with a deli. Oh man, that is good whole food and it's ready to go. I eat right there in the store at the tables. and it's 20% cheaper than fast food as well. Problem solved.

Habit #10: What about cheat days?
Cheat days are days when you can eat anything you want, or a day that you get off the schedule. You are allowed to have a cheat day, but I recommend like one every 30 days until your first 90 days is up. I mean theoretically, on this program, you could eat wedding cake if it's scheduled and portion sized appropriately. On my cheat days, I over eat the chocolate and ice cream or pizza. You can only digest so much at one given time any way. Also, sometimes I am calorie deprived on these days so my body craves any calories it can get, so they might as well be good tasting.

FEMALES

On average, most females require approximately 1200-1300 calories per day when following a healthy weight-loss plan. The following plan is set just shy of 1200 calories. On average, the typical nutrient breakdown per meal should consist of 20% of calories from protein, 60% of calories from carbohydrate, and 20% of calories from fat.

The Machine doesn't run on exercise. It needs high-octane gasoline and quality oil. You must understand that no amount of exercise is going to have a positive effect on your body unless you have proper diet and lifestyle change. The diet is 99.9% of all the results from your training. Whether trying to burn fat, build muscle or create endurance, whatever it is you are trying to do, you need to adjust and schedule your feedings. Scheduling of meals is the most important part of my lifestyle change. I eat every three hours beginning at 6 am when I wake up. Then again at 9am, noon, 3pm, 6pm and 9pm. My largest meal is at noon and nothing after 9pm until I wake at 6am, unless I am in a training camp. Then I add a 1am juice and protein and small snacks in between during the day, when I am burning up to 4,000 calories. Then I repeat the cycle at 6am.

*EXAMPLE of a MACHINE FIT DAILY **HEALTHY MEAL** PLAN #A*

6am : Yogurt, supplements
9am : Scrambled eggs, oatmeal
10:30am : Cottage Cheese (Low Fat is poison, eat the regular one), fruit, peanuts
Noon: Steak, Chicken or Fish, Green Vegetable
3pm : Cottage cheese, fruit, peanuts
4pm: Yogurt
6pm : Steak, Chicken or Fish, green vegetable
9pm : Vegetable Juicer or a fiber rich vegetable

not mandatory
1am: Wake your self up. An additional meal at this time, when training at a high level, will get your metabolism racing. Then back to sleep.

*EXAMPLE of a MACHINE FIT DAILY **HEALTHY MEAL** PLAN #B*

BREAKFAST
1 organic free range egg/ 1 egg white (or, add 1/4 eggbeater/ eggwhite) w/small amount of goat cheese (optional).
1 slice of Ezekiel bread (I like the cinnamon and raisin Ezekiel bread) - from Trader Joes
Or
1/2 cup oatmeal w/ 1 scoop of whey protein your choice of added fruit (blueberries, strawberries, raspberries, etc...)
1 tsp. of ground flax is good to add for additional fiber source and exceptional digestion.

SNACK
Choose one of the following options:
- 1 medium grapefruit and 1 string cheese
- 1/2 homemade turkey wrap with spinach and avocado

LUNCH

(The Largest meal of the day)
3 cups raw spinach
4 oz. of chicken breast
2 oz of peppers, tomatoes, onion and other veggies
3 Tbsp of balsamic dressing

1/2 cup brown rice
Or
Tuna (in water, no sodium) salad
add as many different green veggies as you like
(celery, green onion, assorted peppers, etc...)
1 sweet potato or 1/2 yam
Or
Extra lean ground turkey (prepared in advance) with grilled veggies of your choice
1/2 cup brown rice
salsa if desired

SNACK

Choose one of the following options:
- 1% Greek yogurt (add fruit and/ or granola)
- the other half of your turkey wrap from earlier
- Protein shake

DINNER

(No later than 7:30 pm)
it is always best to have your meals pre-made, but, I always like to cook my dinner fresh.

4 oz chicken breast or a very lean meat
1/2 cup brown rice
1 cup veggies
Or
Balsamic salad from the Lunch menu

LAST MEAL

(No later than 9:00 pm)
I like to end my evening with a dessert-sugar free pudding, a fudge sickle, or a yogurt. I also drink kettle brewed unsweetened Green Tea as an alternative to Water. An ice cold glass is a very satisfying alternative to juice.

*EXAMPLE MACHINE FIT **WEIGHT-LOSS** MEAL PLAN*

BREAKFAST

1 cup yogurt
10 almonds raw, no salt
1/2 cup of egg white
1/2 cup oatmeal plain

SNACK

1/2-3/4 cup egg white
3 oz extra lean ground turkey

LUNCH

1 cup green vegetables
4 oz chicken breast, dry
1/2 cup brown rice

SNACK

1 tbsp flax seed
1 scoop whey protein powder

SNACK

1/2 grapefruit
4 oz extra lean ground turkey

DINNER

10 almonds
1 cup green veggies
1 med salad
2 tbsp of low sugar balsamic

4 oz WHITE meat, chicken or fish - grilled, broiled or BBQ'd

Back in the day, during my professional fighting career, when I first discovered the art of dieting, I was taught by a bio chemist and he taught me to eat every fours hours on a 30/40/30, meaning 30% protein, 40% fat and 30% carbohydrates. After my first meal, I immediately felt the boost of energy. Now it has been updated to eat every three and that ratio is not always a 30/40/30 according to what phase of training you are in. It's almost as if you are just grazing all day long. Also, depending on how overweight you are. Also, calorie restriction is a great way to start this phase off. For instance, phase one, the first 30 days of the process, you will start out with a high protein low carb meal, because you are going to be breaking down and building up, so you will need the proteins. As you enter the second phase, you moderately need less protein and more carbs. The third phase requires higher carbs for energy.

My wife was looking good. She and I were at the gym in Fountain Valley, working out, when we met a new trainer by the name of Brad. It was funny, because for a minute there, she was confusing he and I for the same guy. I guess we kind of looked alike, but he was a bodybuilder, though I didn't hold that against him. He was also a Nutritionist/biochemist.

We befriended Brad and he taught me the significance of eating a complete meal comprised of 30/ 40/ 30: protein, fat, and carbohydrates. It was designed to get my energy from fat that is already in your body, and not carbs. The meals made an immediate difference in my energy levels and athletic performance.

And because she was such a fantastic cook, she prepared the meals and made them even better, like cottage cheese with pineapple and crushed peanuts. Before then, my work out meal was a protein drink followed by a carb drink, all fat cut out of my diet. In retrospect, I don't know how I fell into the bodybuilder trap of no fat, ugh. Lions eat fat and protein and carbs, and they're still muscular, lean, and quick. If eating like that is good enough for a lion, it had to be good enough for me.

Before this, I believed I had to eat a no fat diet. That would get me shredded. Wrong. A lion eats the whole zebra and he is the King. He is ripped and muscular. He eats the Protein, carbs AND the fat. In fact, if you do not eat fat, this will cause your body to hold on to extra fat. That is not optimum. Additionally, a no fat diet over a long period of time is horrible for the cardiovascular system. It tears you up inside and is a leading cause of heart disease.

Fat is also essential for aiding in the slowing of digestion. Every natural protein has fat in it. If a carb is eaten alone, it liquefied and spikes the glycemic index and rushes into the blood stream. Fat slows this down. It's kind of like smearing melted wax over a screen, the stomach lining. It will increase the amount of time it takes to digest your meal.

There are good carbs and bad carbs. Meaning, some carbs digest faster (bad) than others (good). If you hold a handful of steamed white rice in the palm of your hand and hold it under warm water, then squeeze, it liquefied. If you have a handful of chopped green apples and do that, what happens? That's what happens in your stomach.

Dieting for a lifestyle change is not easy and requires a huge amount of motivation and discipline. I have mastered the art of dieting over a lifetime of trial and error. I know what foods work well for me and which do not. For instance, I have food sensitivity to Raspberries. I love them, but they make me light headed, my heart races and it feels like my blood sugar has bottomed out. So, I do not ever eat them. I love peanut butter, apples and beef jerky. It keeps me in an anabolic state. I grow like a weed when I eat that stuff. You will have to discover for yourself, what works and what does not.

It's not cheap to be fit. To eat properly you can spend up to $200 to $400 a week for a single person, and another $100 for any additional. You are going run up a huge food bill. Being fit is not cheap.

Pre and Post workout meals for MMA

As an athlete you should be eating healthy all day, every day. Research has shown that post game/practice nutrition is as equally important as meals eaten prior to competition. There is a slight difference in the meal that is eaten prior to training or games (generally a lighter meal with a good mix of complex carbs) but the meal immediately after activity replenishes your muscles, lessons soreness and quickens recovery. There is a window within an hour following heavy activity. A small serving of protein and a combination of complex carbs seems to be the best way to recover from training. A regular meal can be eaten 1 - 2 hours following the post-practice/ game meal.

The following should help determine good nutritional habits:
1. Eat 4-6 small meals per day

2. Eat 2-4 servings of complex carbs per meal - whole grains, fruits or vegetables
3. Cut out simple carbs from diet - sugar, soda, candy, cakes, white flour
4. Eat protein at every meal - Chicken, turkey, lean red meat, fish, eggs, and reduced fat dairy products.
5. Drink plenty of water
6. Reduce fat intake to less than 25% of your total caloric intake
A. bake, broil or BBQ - meats
B. reduce refined sugars and saturated fats (butter, sour cream)
C. eat healthy fats - omega 3 fatty acids (fish oils), cook with canola oil or olive oil, soy=based foods, health nuts (walnuts, almonds, old fashioned peanut butter)

Let's FEED THE MACHINE.

This is an example of a single day in the life. It's a step-by-step motivational manuscript for you.

OK, it's up to you and no one else to have the discipline and motivation to lose weight and create the desired results. Visualize what you want now.

So, your metabolism has come to a screeching halt and your 50lbs over weight and you have zero energy.

Well, don't panic. It is possible to lose that weight and get your metabolism started again and melt that shit away.

You must believe this will work for best results, for the next 90 days you are committed.

First, begin 20-minute workouts 2-3 times a week of heavy weights, body weight exercises, and or sprinting. This will kick start your metabolism to start searching for calories for a 2-3 day period after each workout.

Second, add 30-minute sessions of walking, jogging or swimming, 3-4 days a week to keep your weight from going up and keeping it down.

Third, you have to schedule and portion control your diet. You must stoke your metabolism first thing when you wake up with a small glass of cold water followed by a bowl of oatmeal and peanut butter. No journal is necessary.

2-3 hours later, eat a small green veggie, an egg or yogurt with a glass of water, quickly, then, move on.

*I will answer any question you have and give you an absolute solution. JohnLober@yahoo.com

2-3 hours later, just as you begin to feel hungry again, hold out 10 or 15 minutes and let your body search for the calories it needs from the fat in your body. That is hunger pain. Then medicate it, or eat again, another small meal. Banana and peanut butter or whatever makes you feel good until lunch whatever time that is, usually noon.

Lunch is the biggest meal of the day. For the first 30 days, it is the size of your fist. Make it a good one.. I am not concerned with what it is, beef, chicken, or fish. Butter and mayonnaise are not your enemies, starving is.

Now, be prepared. Do not get caught without food in 3 hours when you have digested lunch or you are screwed. Save part of your lunch, bring an apple or a string cheese and a handful of nuts. Have something ready for the 3'oclock hour. It is crucial to keeping your fire hot.

Drink water all day long. It's like flushing a toilet with a poop in it. Waste needs to be flushed out of your body frequently. Period.

*No carbonation. No sweeteners and flavored drinks.

Okay, you're working a lot and stressing, but you are being fed enough food to last you every 2-3hours. This will give you confidence that your Machine is running at Optimum calorie burning and your fireplace (metabolism) is running hot.

At this point, we are not really concerned if the

ratios are perfect, fat, carbs and proteins, just that they are all there in every meal.

We would always like to slow down the rate of digestion with fibrous carbs, but when in doubt, just add a tablespoon of peanut butter. That will do the trick. I love peanut butter because it is close to a complete food, but importantly, it has the essential fats that will slow digestion of any carb. The fat will clog up the screen or lining of your stomach.

Processed foods are complete crap and that's why they are cheap and you can get a fucking triple coupon for them. This shit will give you cancer, a fat ass and allergies and all kinds of complications. Stay clear of these.

Now, you should be getting off work soon. You are beat up. Getting cranky because your still adjusting portion sizes, your stomach is hungry and you want to pig out at happy hour. Fuck that! I have good news, you get dinner at 6pm. If you didn't do your exercise after your first meal, or walk at lunchtime, then you have to bust out a fast 20 minutes now.

If your dinners have not been cooked, pre made and Tupperware packed, ready to eat, by you or your personal chef, then this is where I can help you. Drink some water now. Change your clothes and go. Get it done and be ready to eat right when you are finished. You have to do this to spark your fire if it is not a rest day. You get two rest days a week, meaning, you still eat the same, you just do not sweat. One is an active day with a light walk, the other you do not do anything. Both can be non-active if you are in pain. If your not working, eating or training, you are sleeping. if you do not sleep at least 6-8 hours everyday, you are fucked. You will short out your metabolism and it will hold the fat.

You will begin to feel energized within the first three days, you will have aches n pains but fuck it, you are not injured and you are burning fat. Take one Advil. You are allowed to cut back on the workouts to give yourself 3-4 rest days if you think you need to, but keep the feeding schedule.

*If you fuck up, it's OK. Just pick back up where you left off.

Now, the last meal is upon us at 9 o'clock. This is what makes or breaks every mutherfucker that "diets". It should be a liquid shake or something like a cucumber with hot sauce. I don't care what it is, just keep it small and sensible, and preferable fibrous. Your guts will squeeze fiber like ringing a towel and burn calories while you sleep. Do not eat anything else after 9 until you wake up. This is when you fast. Your body eats the fat up in your body, searching for calories in your fat. You have to be asleep for this to happen. Period. You will wake up feeling skinnier after fasting. Now, back to the top and break the fast. Drink some cold water, then put any food you can get on your tongue. Stoke the fire. Feed the Machine or whatever you call it. You will have awesome results in 90days. Then we will dial it in and do it again, making it a lifestyle, for higher intensity during workouts.

It was time to feed the Machine properly.

3. Training vs Working out

To be successful you need to workout. When you go to the gym you are doing a workout. You may do this everyday, waking up early and going in before work or at lunch break. Sometimes you count how many times you worked out. Occasionally it may be twice a day. You usually try your best during these mundane exercises and hopefully you get a quick nap in between sessions, usually not.

This is different from training, which requires management and logging of your daily workouts and diet lifestyle on a daily, weekly and monthly basis. Training is paying attention to your precise modification of your caloric and nutritional intake, the amount of sleep your getting and the amount of stress you are placing on your body. Training is focused on a specific athletic event or goal in your program with Optimum Performance Levels maximized. It is periodized in intensity to a peak in performance. You are programming yourself for success and cycling the intensities to peak at a specific goal.

"Train smarter, not harder."-JL

Mixed Martial Arts training is becoming extremely popular and will result in total body fitness and toning. I highly recommend the P90x or UFCfit programs for durability in everyone and the CrossFit for a more optimum performance and general fitness in athletic training.
http://youtu.be/NuqHv-bjL-A
General rule of thumb, lifting heavy weights will increase your metabolism and keep it burning for two to three days after each session. Walking, Jogging, Swimming, cycling and rowing will keep

your weight down when performed consistently with proper eating.

Sport specific training, like Jiu-jitsu, cardio kickboxing and football, will build necessary technical skills, but need the supplemental conditioning programs to reach Optimum Performance Levels.

Any program you decide to participate in will have a desired effect and a plateau at a 90-day period. It should be scaled back in intensity or changed to a different system to overcome plateaus in order to progress to Optimum Performance levels in MMA.

There are other specific training concepts that can enhance OPT. Plyometrics will increase power by adding speed with strength to agility training. Bands are excellent for keeping pressure off joints and building strength and balance. Balance exercises are extremely beneficial to adding to strength by stabilizing joints. I use a large ball and a balance disc for my balance regiment. Tabatas are my favorite for explosive conditioning. I personally almost never do the same workout twice. My muscles have memory and after three sessions on a specific system I am trained up and ready to roll.

High intensity exercise for a short duration of a minimum of 15-20 minutes will burn sugar for energy and break down muscle. Low intensity exercise for a longer duration of a minimum of 30 minutes will use fat as energy. In fact, it is better if you do not sweat because it is a more efficient manner of burning fat and losing weight.

Does Heat and vigorous exercise help you sweat out toxins?
You aren't likely to purify your body of much of anything by sweating, whether in a hot yoga class or

sizzling sauna, because all that's in perspiration is water, salt, and a smattering of electrolytes and essential nutrients. Sweat glands sit in the skin and aren't connected to other systems in the body, so it makes no sense that they would eliminate waste. The only role of perspiration is to keep you cool. The body does a pretty good job of getting rid of what it doesn't need, largely through the liver, kidneys, and digestive tract. There's nothing special you have to do to help, other than eat well, stay hydrated, and keep fit so those organs can function properly.

I spent a period of three years during my early twenties, before mixed martial arts, when I specifically focused on only strength lifts, like bench press, over head press, squat and deadlifts. I had an amazing strength mentor as my first trainer. Sulby Prince Strength. One of my earliest role models was Sulby Prince from MiddleSex, England. He was a 280-pound body builder, criminal and addict. He looked like a Bart Simpson hulk with a bleached white flat top and always wearing his polarized prescription sunglasses. His accent was a thick baritone English slang. He moved to Huntington Beach for the weather. He said England weather was too depressing. He hated the company of drunk people and hated feeling tired. He would slam cocaine or Nubian, a synthetic morphine, or anything he could to combat this. He had this mammoth chiseled physique with these three calloused injection sites. He had one on each enormous arm and one on his calf. He would wake up, slam that shit then suck up water out of a glass with the empty syringe then purge the blood out of the syringe so he could re use it. Sulby was Mr. California in '95 and a World's Strongest Man. I heard from an ex-roommate that he actually drank his urine to recycle his steroids.

Up until I met Sulby, I was just working out with my Dad, just priming the charge for the real results. We bought Joe Weider protein powder in five pound bags from local nutrition shop and would split it up in large Tupperware containers. We bought two gallons of milk and two dozens of eggs every three days from Costco and every Wednesday we would religiously eat all you can eat lasagna at the Italian restaurant. Calories are like socks, you cant have too many.

Before too long, I was training with Sulby every morning at 7 am sharp. He had just done three months in OCJ for falling asleep in his car with the needle still in his arm. He was a very intense dude with a very strict set of life rules. If you were late or didn't show up at all, he would immediately cut you for life from the SP team. He didn't have many friends and hated my girlfriend .

Sulby was in his 30's but if you asked him he was 28, and had been 28 for about seven years now. That was funny to me. After going "Hollywood" on an all niter, when he would show up to train the strippers. He would have his headphones on with the cord just tucked in his pocket, no Walkman. Sometimes, he would just call the payphone on the wall and have the women in a line so he could tell them what to do. And, he was the one that gave me the inspiration to actually LIVE in the gym, A Gym Rat, for saving time of course.

Before too long I learned what training to failure was all about. Pushing through the pain barrier. I suppose it was really tough to normal folk. I loved it. I was ringing out my T-shirt at the end of the 7 -10 am workouts. Soon, I saw incredible strength gains and with that comes size. Without any drugs.

Sulby would lift the heaviest, most mammoth amount of weight he possibly could every single rep and set. Making it count. I wanted to do the same. He could load the leg press up to nearly a thousand pounds and deep press it with a single leg. It was incredible to watch. He was screaming and yelling. I learned the difference between strict muscling and leveraging or cheating the weight up. My favorite lift was the deadlift which was a compound exercise and the vertical leg press which I could load heavier than a bar squat.

"Everyone is a junkie junior." according to SP before too long he was injecting me with testosterone to increase my recovery rate. Powerhouse gym on Main Street was like a church with a lot of regulars. I met Kimo, the UFC legend, there and I met Todd through SP. Todd was the largest steroid, and anything else, dealer in OC at the time so those two had a lot in common. They ate thousands of calories, dozens and dozens of hard-boiled eggs, gallons of milk and Joe weirder protein powder, and a lot of trips to all you can eat lasagna nights at Nick's Pizza D' Oro. The two of them were experimenting with the HGH at the time among the regular cornucopia, including Nubian and other street drugs. They both were topping 295lbs of ripped muscle and strong as a hulk.

So, Todd finally gets me to dabble with Nubain.

The pain barrier was what I was battling. Battling through. We would start off with bench press let's say. I would load the bar up to what I thought my max lift was and with a spot from Sulby, I would do one or two reps then rack it without moving my hands from the bar while Sulby stripped the weight a little at a time. Then I would do six or seven more reps then rack it again and Sulby stripped the bar a little more. As many of these sets as it took to get to just the bar and I would squeeze out what little strength I had left in me. Day in, day out every lift, every rep was my max effort until I failed daily. Boy, that hurt so good. I could literally ring my shirt out and fill a small bucket with sweat.

My word for strength was "UP." If I said the word UP, I could lift an extra 100 lbs, or at least it felt like it. The heaviest lift I could record as a personal record, was a 650 pound deadlift at 202lbs. Later I would switch to lifting the back end of my truck for convenience.

We implemented the Mike Menzer or Dorian Yates type of going to failure type strength training, on a three on one off schedule. If the day off happened to be a Friday I was allowed to take Saturday off also, and boy did I need it.

Powerhouse Strength Schedule:

DAY 1   Monday : Chest/ Back
DAY 2   Tues :   Shoulders/ Arms
DAY 3   Wed :   Legs
DAY 4   Thursday : REST
DAY 5   Friday :   Chest/ Back
DAY 6   Saturday : Shoulders/ Arms
DAY 7   Sunday :   Legs
Day 8   Monday : REST
Day 9   Tuesday : Chest/ Back
Day 10   Wed :   Shoulders/ Arms
Day 11   Thursday : Legs
Day 12   Friday :   REST
Day 13   Saturday : REST

This was my foundation for my Herculean strength. For the most part I did it without the aid of steroids, so I kept 90% of the gains. I earned them without "cheating". I mean I dabbled with the D Bol earlier, but I wouldn't even take an Advil before a workout prior to meeting SP. But hey, if your not cheating, your not trying, so next came the Parabolin. Parabolin is a steroid that didn't aromatize and gave me some serious size and strength. I wasn't genetically a Bodybuilder, I was built to be strong. Did a couple short cycles with that and fuck, there wasn't enough weight in the gym after long. Then came the Nubain! Then came a dark fucking slide, but I was big and happy, or so I thought.

I discontinued all that drug use shortly after Sulby flew back to England where he was from and became hooked on Brazilian Jiu Jitsu. I was finished with the strength workouts, cut them back to once a week and completely jumped into technical training and grappling. After a lot of craziness, SP went back to England to avoid a 3 year suspended sentence after riding pops bike through a stop sign. He handed me a fat sack of blue and yellow Valium. I never saw him again. He died of a heart attack 20 years later, RIP.

The early UFC events were the most incredible spectacles I had ever witnessed in my entire violent lifestyle to this point. It was an evil circus of death and impending doom fueled by extreme alcohol and drug abuse. It was like a trigger for me to indulge. I instantly fell in lust. It meant I could be as inappropriate as I wanted to be and get away with it.

My first grappling training buddy was Chris. He was an ex bodybuilder with a short stocky blonde gremlin look with a raspy deep voice and huge grippers (hands). We met at UFC 6 in Casper, Wyoming. Todd and I were there to watch Tank Abbotts UFC debut in Casper, Wyoming. I met Leon Spinks, Ken Shamrock and Dan Severn. It was great. Tank and his crew, the guy that is Tito's coach later in the story, were raising hell everywhere they went and had everyone on edge. Beating people up in elevators, inappropriateness, vandalizing shit, etc.. They were violent drunk assholes. (Important later for the Tito frank fight) I was looking forward to the after party. Chris and I agreed if Tank won the final we were not going to attend the party because there would be some real bullshit going on then. Well, Tank kills Johnny Matua with a thunderous punch that sent Johnny into a de-cerebrate seizure and completely detached his brain from his spine. It was awesome. A life changing experience for Johnny too. I had only seen Samoans do that to white dudes at parties. Sucker punches and shit like that, they were assholes, so I instantly became a fan of Tanks for fucking that guy up like that. It gave me confidence I could do it too. I am not a fan of the guy that uses the sucker punch. Well, there was an incredible altitude in Wyoming and in an unbelievable 30-minute fight with Oleg Takterov, Tank lost the decision and would probably have to go to the hospital. Oleg did, Tank did not, but that still meant that we could go to the after party. We jumped up and down and went hard into celebrating. Lots of celebrities, like John Wayne Bobbit, the guy who cock his dick cut off by his girlfriend. I got so drunk, I think I pissed in some girls purse, the mystery pisser strikes again.

Drunk as skunks and having a good time back at the room, Chris and I end up grappling. He grabs my head from the guard. He had a couple months on me with the Jiu-jitsu. I had no training at this time. So, he is choking me with the guillotine from his guard and I start pounding his ribs. He let go and said I tapped.
"Yah, right!' I said. "You let go because I was beating your body mutherfucker!"

When we got home, he and I got together at the karate school that would later hold the ground fighting tournaments at, and we would train. Then to the Thunder center.

I came home after leaving my job with Pepsi and told my girlfriend I was quitting my job so I could do my plan, laser focus on being on PPV and being the world champion. I was that confident.

Chris was in a Kimono and Punchy, my girlfriends little brother, and I were in sweat pants and T shirts. I was tapping him out now. He was pissed and stopped training with me. He did give me a pretty sweet Cauliflower ear as a parting gift though. From laying on my face and twisting my ear up in his Kimono when he switched crossed sides. It popped and I had to learn how to drain it with these left over syringes I had.

Punchy and I ended up at Ken Gabrielson's full time. Chris had worn out his welcome there. Chris would go from instructor to instructor and would talk a little shit at each place and it always got back to Ken. It was a small community at the time. He would learn a little here and a little there until he finally ended up traveling to Brazil for a while. The Brazilians call this kind of guy, a Creote'. A nomad. And they were the worst kind of student to the Brazilians because it was a threat to their business. They were not true to any instructor. Money is a Brazilians god. They would destroy traditional BJJ structure, and just be bad for business.

Chris and I realized early off that the specialist was not going thrive in the fight world or even as a sportsman. So, we trained everywhere. Remember Bo Knows...the Nike saying. Cross training was coming up at this time and we just applied it to the martial arts first, the strength training, then the cardio. Everybody eventually had to become a cross trainer to excel at the new sport to be a complete fighter. The important thing was giving respect to your roots. Everyone gave me the respect or I took it.

"To be a champion, you need to challenge yourself at one thing, at a high level, every day."-JL

Change and challenge is the key to success. It applies to training. If I only did one type of workout for five years day in day out, there would be no reason for my body to change or adapt to any challenges. So, I mix it up to increase growth and OPL's.

After a short stay in Prison in '05, I made a decision to create something larger than just me, (see my other book Memoirs of a Machine: Inside the Mind of aCagefighter)

Team MACHINE MMA Worldwide. It is a global concept. These are my Training Objectives:

Instructor: Coach John Lober
Assistant Instructors: Joe Flahavan & Jojo Guillaume
Academy: Team Machine MMA
Atlanta, California, Hawaii
Phone: 714 975-4850
email: JohnLober@yahoo.com

Objective:
Train. Fight. Win.

Kicking hurts and Grappling is a tough sport. All sessions are designed to develop fundamental skills, techniques and tactics in Brazilian Jiu-Jitsu, Clinch,

Boxing and Muay Thai Competition. Workouts and drills will be held at the Team Machine Academy as well as other fitness facilities. You are going to burn a lot of calories on your quest for optimum athletic output and you will become proficient in a huge array of martial art skills necessary for competition or you will just become more durable with this positive lifestyle change.

As a prospective member of Team MACHINE there are certain responsibilities you will be held accountable for. These are set in place to create consistency and effectiveness for upcoming competition. Each athlete is expected to do the following:

Represent TEAM MACHINE Athletics in a positive manner.
Treat yourself and others with courtesy and respect.
Be drug free.

DESIRE, DEDICATION, DISCIPLINE, DETERMINATION.
Responsibilities:

Be on time to Practice . Tardiness is not acceptable behavior. If an emergency or illness arises, please notify Coach Lober in person, by phone or email before the absence occurs.
Injuries occur in Martial Arts training and you assume all risks. Our goal is to minimize these injuries through proper instruction of techniques and controlled sparring.
The transmission of communicable skin conditions is a major concern. Proper hygiene is important including properly trimmed nails on hands and feet. To minimize ringworm, etc.. It is essential to properly clean the mat before and after practice. Everyone is required to keep the facility clean. The Academy is properly cleaned after every session. Remove your

shoes at the door. No running in the grappling room. No horseplay on the mats. Your Gi is mandatory and must be washed after each practice. No hair gel. Becoming a great athlete does not start with skills. It starts with the love of the sport. The most important aspect of exceptional athletes is their drive, which is closely related to passion. Training out side the structure of practices and meets shows the real interest in being successful - competing and winning!

Your words and actions are the most important things you own; no one can take those away. Commitment to Team MACHINE is no different. There are two rules that you will need to follow: #1. Be on time and #2. Always give your best. Committing to play on a team means that you have entered a verbal contract to work as hard as you can to help your teammates and yourself to improve, to compete and win.

If you step on the mat doubting if you can win, then you should expect to lose. If you don't think you can improve your skills, then you won't. Great athletes believe that every practice is a chance to improve. Without belief you will have to depend on luck and luck loses to belief every time.

All practices will begin with a warm-up routine and this is the time that your focus needs to narrow down to one thing, Jiu-Jitsu. No distractions! All your energy and effort is directed towards the coaches, your teammates and yourself in an effort to be the best athlete on the best team.

The will to win, there is no substitute. Competing is not just restricted to tournaments. Competing in every practice against your teammates and challenging yourself to do your best in every phase of the workout. Tapping does not discourage a winner it only motivates them to work harder.

Great athletes inspire their teammates. The way they practice, the way they compete and the level of commitment they bring to a team makes other team members work harder. One's inspiration is an infectious attitude that can bring an entire team together while raising he level of competitiveness.

TEAM MACHINE CONCEPTS.

1. Fighter / Martial Artist = DISCIPLINE, Determination, Dedication
and Desire.
2. Approach JKD with the idea of mastering the will. Forget about winning and losing; forget about pride and pain. Let your opponent graze your skin and you smash into his flesh; let him smash into your flesh and you fracture his bones; let him fracture your bones and you take his life! Do not be concerned with your escaping safely- lay your life before him!
3. It is a way of life.
4. While being trained, the student is to be active and dynamic in Every Way. But in actual combat, his mind must be calm and not at all disturbed. He must feel as if nothing critical is happening. When he advances, his steps should be light and secure, his eyes NOT fixed and glaring insanely at the enemy. His behavior should not be in any way different from his everyday behavior, no change taking place in his expression, nothing betraying the fact that he is engaged in mortal combat.
5. It is indeed difficult to see the situation simply - our minds are very complex - and it is easy to teach one to be skillful, but it is difficult to teach him his own attitude, angle of approach.
6. This nameless art calls for complete mastery of techniques, developed by reflection within the soul.
7. The art is an expression of life and transcends both time and space.
8. The essence of fighting is the art of moving. Footwork will always beat any kick or punch.

4. Running on empty

Now get ready to break all the rules I just explained to you. I was coming off a year or two lay off and I was out of shape. My body snapped back into shape quickly, training twice a day at a high level for 30 days, but I needed something else to enhance my state of mind. I had primed the charge and I was ready to go to the OPL. I had a case of AAA grade beef from my sponsor in the fridge at the gym where I was staying, but instead of eating right when I woke up at 5 am like I had been, I would put my shoes on and hit the street for a 5-10 mike march. Fasting the entire time, until I got back to the gym for grappling. Boy was I angry and driven. I was training with guys 10 years younger than me and stronger too now, but I was destroying them again, and fat was melting off my mid section faster than ever and my strength was back. Then I would load up on AAA ground beef patties from the Beef Palace for lunch and dinner. I was at OPL again.

Fasting like this introduced nutritional stress, not by restricting total calories, but by cycling periods of fasting or under-eating for over 12 hours—or sometimes 16—a day. I was triggering stress response agents that were eating all the bad shit out of my body like the Cavemen used to do. Stress protein, heat shock proteins, certain kinds of enzymes, and anti-inflammatory and immune molecules that practically search and destroy every weak element in your body were released and it put me in a state of mind that was driven to Optimum Performance Levels. And besides, this saved me a ton of money on my food bill.

Eating every two hours or eating six meals a days, however, isn't stressful on your body. Following a regular schedule and avoiding hunger is the opposite, but necessary.

5. Shutting Down

"A "normal" person is one that goes to sleep at the same time and wakes up at the same time every day."-JL

I used to sleep 12 to 16 hours a day. As I got older I only need 8 hours, and when I am training at a high level I require a 45-minute mid day nap, especially in between training sessions. The room should be dark, cool and noise free, besides any type of sports hypnosis or meditation you are playing on the iPod. Recovery is the most important factor to OP than diet and training together. It is when we are rebuilding ourselves back, stronger. If I walked into the gym and felt I couldn't give a 100%, I would pick up my bag and go home and sleep. If you are in a constant state of being catabolic, breaking down, you will over train, get weak and sick, and go backwards with no results. Active rest days when you do light exercise with no sweating are ideal for recovery.

"Eat for strength, Sleep for speed."-JL

Optimum Health and Fitness and the common cold.

Please listen to me. This is very important to your Health and Fitness.
The Flu is not just a cloud that comes over us and we get sick. It is around us 24/7 and there are three factors that lower your immune system and make you susceptible to getting sick.
1. STRESS. Mental stress of a demanding job, deadlines, bosses, etc... Physical stress. Training like your on the biggest Loser, or two a days at Crossfit and just pounding yourself into the ground to failure with every workout, cutting weight, etc....

2. POOR DIET. Not only eating processed crappy foods with little nutritional values, but also not eating enough. When you sweat, you are sweating out the essential vitamins and Minerals mandatory for your recovery. Eating food and drinking water will not replace this soup of minerals you are sweating out, thus your recovery will be hindered. 3. LACK OF SLEEP. You have to get your 6 to 8 every night.

6. A Daily Journal

Nicole Flores is my latest and most enthusiastic client as of late. She is a 36 year old, Hispanic female. 4' 11" with 2 kids and currently weighs 177 lbs.. Nicole has been fit in the past, but feels she has let herself go and now realizes she is 50 lbs overweight. She has had significant success since beginning the program to Optimize her nutrition in just the first 60 days. She started a new career at the same time she began this journey. Nicole has a Masters degree from University of Phoenix and I believe this was a contributing factor. It helped her to journal on a daily basis as she reported to me daily. I held her accountable for her work as I coached her over a long distance via email and phone. Following are her journal entries to help you as you begin to Optimize your Health. Note that the significant thing in her journals is the comments on how she feels. This is important in finding your niche. And later will help you remember what works well for you and what does not.

Nicole's Journal:

Day 1:
5:20 wake up
5:25
    16 oz. Room temperature H2o
5:45
    1 nonfat yoplait yogurt strawberry shortcake
5:55
    2 cups black coffee w/ 1/4 cup 2% milk
9:15
    3 strawberries
    5 raw almonds
12:15 Lunch
3:15

Green smoothie:
2 cups spinach
I cup frozen berries
1 cup almond milk
1 Tbsp almond butter

Prep dinner:
Homemade veggie soup
I cup 6pm

15 min spinning

1 hour yoga

9pm
1 scoop protein powder with almond milk

Day 2

6am
Water
gogurt

9am
1/2 cup dry Quaker oats
tsp. almond slivers
cranberries
1/2 tsp. honeyWater

12pm
4 strawberry w/ peanut butter

3pm
tuna (.5 tsp mayo) salad w/ 1/4 avocado
balsamic vinegar& lite cesar dressing

6pm peanut butter
celery and carrot in chicken broth

9pm peanut butter w/ banana

I have been able to eat on schedule. I was at the baseball field at noon so I had my big lunch at 3pm. It worked out good since I had oatmeal for breakfast.I feel good , not hungry; right when I start to feel hungry its time to eat in 15 min anyway. It's really amazing how that's been working out that way... I'm feeling soar in my shoulders. Maybe from the weights earlier today. . No biggie. But its been nice to recover from the cardio rat race.

Day 3:
5:00 am
> Water
> yogurt
> Water

820am
> 1/4 cup dry oatmeal cinnamon,
> 1/2 tsp honey
> 1/2 tsp dry nondairy creamer
> 1 Tbsp almond slivers dried cranberries.

830 spin class
> Water!

1130am
> 6 raw almonds
> 1 apple
> Water

250pm
> sauteed in olive oil tilapia 2cups spinach
> 1 cup broccoli
> Water

615pm
> 1/2 avocado
> 4oz fish
> 2 shrimps
> vegetable soup
> Ice tea

10pm
> banana
> peanut butter
> Water

Woke up early today. Dumb cat lol had to made a shitload of spaghetti for my son's potluck this am anyway and then get to spin class before it started..then yay lots of fun with jumpers at the park and a bunch of kids running around! Oh yes and NOT visiting the potluck food table! Brought my own snacks!! Yesterday in yoga I felt so strong in my poses, I was dripping sweat. Then she had us doing some really deep hamstring stretches I mean really deep I thought my arm was going to fall off from holding my leg over my head for so long! Today at spin class it was tough but I felt powerful. I did 10.8 miles in 36 minutes. I got a good sweat going felt a little winded at first but id rather push myself good and honest for 35 min than coast for 70, make my one cardio day count!

Day 4:

615am

    Water
    Yogurt
    Coffee
    1/8 cup almond milk unsweetened

910am

    1/4 cup oats boiled in Water, 1tsp dry nondairy creamer
    1 / 2 tsp honey
    1 Tbsp almond slivers cranberries
    Water

100pm 5oz steak 1/3 cucumber, 1/4 avocado, shredded carrots
    1.5 cups romaine lettuce
    1 / 4 tomato
    2 Tbsp lite Cesar dressing

430

    1.5 Cup cottage cheese
    7 raw almonds
    1 cup pineapple

620pm

    1 cup broccoli
    peanut butter

8pm
yoga
915pm

    banana

peanut butter

Yes love my new job just learning and taking it all in! They have hot/ cold water and refrigerator so I'm good! Gonna bring a cutting board and stock the fridge. I'm moving in lol. I did a relaxing yoga stretch at home and some plank and ab work.
Day 5:

630 am
- Water
- yogurt
- Coffee with
- 1 /4 cup almond milk

930
- Oatmeal with
- tsp of dry nondairy creamer 1/2 tsp honey
- 1 Tbsp dry fruit and nuts
- Water

1pm
- 4oz tilapia sautéed in olive oil and 2 cups spring mix
- carrot shreds 1 Tbsp lite cesar dressing
- Green tea

4pm
- peach and peanut butter

7pm
- 1 cup broccoli w peanut butter

930   brisk walk
10pm   1/4 cup cottage cheese 5 raw almonds
1.5 cups fresh pinapple

Today was fantastic I could feel my body searching for calories, now that I'm well aware. I am realizing people eat what's in front of them. If you don't prepare and feed your body, you starve yourself and get desperate. So you will eat donuts or whatever is in front of you especially if it's free. I see this happening all day long at work and the kids games
I have some off site training on Monday and the will feed me a healthy lunch like chicken salad but I will have to pack snacks.
I had a bit of a headache today stress dehydration info overload at work or combination of everything. It was nice to end the day with a nice walk in the evening.

Day 6

730
- Water
- yogurt

830
spin class
- Water

1040pm
- yogurt
- Water

120pm
- hardboiled egg
- orange
- Water

420pm
- peach
- peanut butter

700pm
- 5 grapes
- 2 strawberries

900pm

8oz fish soup with vegetables (carrots, celery, tomatoes and onions)
3/4 avocado plain
ice tea.
Water

Rocked it in spin class! Rode for 40 minutes then called it quits. Didn't want to overdo it! Was able to keep my watts at my body weight and keep my rpm at 80-110. Pretty awesome it felt good to pull my body weight with ease. It's really nice to have people make comments about me looking slimmer. Did well at the baby shower then bbq today. I didn't find any good meat protein at the party so I had tilapia fish soup for dinner. Overate a bit and felt too full. Have not had that feeling in awhile and it did not feel good. But I'm glad I did because it reminded me of why eating smaller portions is important!!!

Day 7

720

    Water
    yogurt
    Started feeling hungry about

945

    Water

1020

    oatmeal
    dried fruit and nuts with honey and dry nondairy creamer
    Water

115pm

    4oz tilapia
    1 cup romaine shredded carrots 1/4 tomato Tbsp Cesar dressing

350   started feeling hungry

4pm

    yogurtWater

7pm
- Spinach salad
- brussel sprouts
- strawberries
- raspberry vinaigrette

9pm
- weights

10pm
- banana
- peanut butter

Definitely felt hungry after my workout tonight. I was also really hungry when I woke up this morning probably because of my intense yoga class last night and I stood up pretty late..I was hungry after lunch maybe I did not eat enough. I drink water throughout the day so I don't pay attention especially when im busy. But I will try to be more aware so I can make sure I'm eating enough and not waiting too long in between meals.

Day 8

645
- Water
- Yogurt
- Coffee black
- Water

10am
- Strawberry
- almonds
- Water

1245pm
- 7 oz chicken
- 3/4 avocado
- 2 cups lettuce
- 1/2 2 salsa grilled pepper and onion
- Water

4pm
- 3 strawberry

        4 almonds
        Water

7pm
        banana w peanut butter

815pm
        yogurt
        Water

845-10:15pm workout

10:30pm
        2cups spinach and 1celery and 1 carrot sautéed in olive oil

Ending my 3rd week I have lost 6.6 lbs! Been feeling a little more hungry today. I hope I can make it through my fast on Sunday!! It was interesting to take my time and do weights at the gym. I've never done a weight workout at the gym because there are too many people there and it's sort of embarrassing. Tonight it was fairly empty so I got to take my time and use the bench for my chest presses and a 40 lbs weight for deadlifts while looking in the mirror to make sure my form was good. I also did 3 sets of10 lower leg lifts. I was able to get in some floor ab work then did 30 min low impact cardio. Fun workout!

Day 9

720
        Water
        Yogurt
        Black coffee

1020
        Banana
        Peanut butter
        Green tea

1245
        not hungry much but my lunch got switched due to training
        6oz Grilled chicken
        2 cups romaine lettuce
        2 Tbsp Cesar dressing

　　　　shredded carrots
　　　　Water
4pm
　　　　banana w peanut butter
　　　　Water
　　　　Chores
7pm
　　　　banana w peanut butter
　　　　Water
　　　　Got hungry about 845pm
　　　　Did more chores
10pm
　　　　yogurt

　　　　Got hungry about 1115

I notice I get hungry before bed and right before dinner. I think I may
need to add more fibrous foods and that will help. Today was a bit crazy
for my schedule so my food menu was kept simple. Easy. I also realize I get hungry after I work out or do activities. I will try and incorporate more vegetables tomorrow. As I start week four it is nice to feel my clothes looser. Although I have not lost the 6 - 8lbs that a typical person might have lost by now I can feel that I have almost lost a dress size or two and that is fine for me!

Day 10
7am
　　　　Water
　　　　yogurt
1030am
　　　　Oatmeal with dried fruit almond slivers &
　　　　non dairy creamer with honey
1pm
　　　　5oz salmon in olive oil
　　　　2 cups mustard
　　　　turnip greens

        kale
        carrots
        1 Tbsp cesar dressing

4pm

        Pineapple chunks with 5 almonds

645

        banana with peanut butter

945pm

        nopales cactus scrambled with eggs
        spinach tomato and salsa

Feeling great! The fast was not a problem physically. I knew as long as I kept my brain busy I would be just fine. I watched a movie read a chapter of a good book did a bunch or chores did yoga and went to the grocery store to prepare my dinner. It wasn't bad at all. I find the only thing I crave is pasta for some reason oh and donuts lol but its all good I'm very determined!!!!

Day 11

7am

        Water
        Yogurt
        Coffee
        coconut milk

1040am

        1/2 cup cooked oatmeal
        1/2 tsp honey
        2 tsp almonds dried cranberries
        1 tsp dry nondairy creamer

1pm

        1/2 cup boiled chicken
        2 cups iceberg lettuce
        1/4 cup avocado
        2 slices cucumber
        2 slices tomato
        1 tsp tapatio

4pm

        banana
        peanut butter

7pm
> 6 strawberry
> 1 tsp cottage cheese
> 1/8 cup tuna

Abs shredder workout Walk 30 min
10pm
> broccoli & cauliflower sautéed in olive oil

1am
> 1/2 cup coconut milk
> 1 cup frozen peaches and pineapple
> 1 tsp almond butter

Kicking ass and taking names! Didn't bat an eyelash to pass up cake at work today. Yesterday at my training there were donuts muffins etc. It's like whatever. Found myself glancing at them for a moment but its like there's no way I even want that shit! Its weird even funny to think about how determined I am! Was so busy kicking ass at work today ALMOST didn't have time for my snack! But heck no I made the time to stop and walk away for a moment! Even if I had to eat my oatmeal and finish it 20 min later. The ab workout was awesome love it!!!

Nice relaxing walk to clear the mind at the end of the day with my 14 yr old son. Magically zen- better than therapy or any drug!

Day 12

7am
> Water
> yogurt
> Coffee with 1 / 2 cup coconut milk

10am
> 1/2 cup cooked oatmeal
> 1 tsp almond slivers & dried cranberries
> 1 tsp dry nondairy creamer 1/2 tsp honey
> Water

115pm
> Tuna (1/2 can with 1 Tbsp olive oil mayo) salad

2 cups swiss chard, turnip & mustard greens, kale shredded carrots &1 celery stalk
Green tea
Water

340pm

almonds

4pm

1 tsp cottage cheese
5 strawberries
Water

7pm

banana w / peanut butter

8pm
Workout

Water

10pm

3 cups iceberg & romaine lettuce garden salad
2 Tbsp Italian
2 Tbsp ranch dressing
4 slices tomato

Yesterday was my Friday night and I knew the gym would be empty so I took advantage of the weight room. I feel energized and positive at work. Its like I'm mentally making a great decision with my life and it permeates throughout every aspect. I had a long conversation with a girl I work with who is very beautiful inside and out. She is at 310 lbs. She's frustrated and has so many digestive issues. I think I was able to help her and educate her a bit about my own journey. My only hope was to plant a tiny seed that her success is possible too. On to the 4th of July where I will be surrounded by hotdogs hamburgers sweets and ALCOHOL! My plan is that I'm the DD so I wont drink. I am gonna leave late to the party so I can have my hearty lunch and take some nuts and fruit for the party to enjoy!

Day 13
7am
    3oz steak
    2 eggs
    Black coffee
    Water
10am Small green apple
    with peanut butter
    Water
1pm
    8oz Salmon chili
    broccoli
    Water
4 pm
    broccoli
    Peanut butter
7pm
    chicken spinach salad with vinegar and ranch
    tomato cucumber olives pepperoncini
10pm
    Peanut butter

Ugh I did not even see your email until like 10pm. Crazy day at work and home. I will do a heavy workout tonight. Any suggestions??

Day 14
6am
    banana
    peanut butter
    Black coffee
9pm
    yogurt
1pm
    8oz steak
    mustard
    greens kale
    Cesar dressing
    2 strawberries
    1/4 avocado

4pm
    sm green apple
    peanut butter

7pm
    yogurt

Workout

10pm
    nopales cactus
    1/16 avocado
    salsa
    2 eggs
    olive oil

1am
    yogurt

Felt a lot better after my workout and getting back on schedule. Heck of a last few days... ready for tomorrow! Gonna do another similar workout tomorrow... but I'll work abs shoulders and biceps.

Day 15

8am
    Water
    Yogurt
    Coffee
    1 / 2 cup unsweetened almond milk

11am
    1/2 cup oatmeal
    almond milk
    almonds
    butter
    cinnamon

145pm
    8 oz. chicken
    cabbage
    onion
    carrots
    broccoli
    lettuce
    dressing

330pm
> yogurt
> cherries

600pm
> romaine lettuce
> cilantro
> dressing
> peanuts

Let the fast begin. Definitely felt my diet progress during this yoga class I feel lighter when in plank and chatarunga and less bulky in my oblique when I do a twisted pose. I really feel like I can twist further as my love handles melt away even my boyfriend noticed there is less to hold onto! Lol I felt good about my last few meals. Drank lots of water and had some herbal tea before bed.

Day 16

Fast all day
> Water
> herbal tea
> black coffee
> 1 cup Coffee
> half & half

615pm
> veggie chili
> 1/ 2 cup cooked lean ground beef
> 1/8 cup crushed tomato
> 3 Tbsp. corn
> 1 cup mushrooms
> 1.25 cups squash
> salt & pepper

815
weights
915pm
> 1 orange
> greek yogurt
> Honey

It felt good to have a nice day to fast I had some errands to run all morning and then to the spa for beatification. It was nice to know that I put the majority of the day into myself. It made me feel so complete and I had some nice reflection time. My thoughts are focused and I'm feeling the rewards of making good choices. I'm also rewarded in my new profession. I would have never imagined my success in life would come from staffing. And yet it's like I found my calling. Helping people find jobs and put food on the table is so fulfilling. My passion and purpose in life is to help people and I know now why God has given me this opportunity: to help others find their purpose and give them the confidence to make good choices. Its like everything makes sense. Overall awesome day. So blessed!

Day 17

2am

    spoonful of peanut butter

730

    Water
    yogurt
    Coffee
    half & half

1030am

    oatmeal
    almond slivers
    dried cranberries honey
    Green tea
    Water

1pm

    6oz chicken salad romaine spinach
    Iceberg lettuce
    Strawberries
    1 tsp sunflower seeds
    1/2 tsp crumbled blue cheese
    Apple balsamic dressing
    Water

430pm

Nectarine peanuts

7pm

brussel sprouts sauteed in olive oil

10pm

orange
yogurt
honey

Day 18

7am

Water
banana
peanut butter
Coffee
half & half
Water

10am

orange
almonds
Water

1pm

6oz ground chicken
iceberg lettuce salad
chili
lemongrass vinegar cilantro
Water

4pm

peanuts
yogurt
2 orange slices

6pm

peanuts

8pm
yoga

Water

9pm

broccoli w peanut butter
Water

Wow I watched myself doing yoga during my class today. In some poses I almost didn't recognize myself I've really trimmed down in my waist I can see it in my face and neck too. Its great to know I'm making progress. I also know my most stubborn places will go last but I'm not discouraged one bit. I'm excited to keep going and to continue kicking ass at work and in my workouts!

Day 19

7am

    Water
    yogurt
    Coffee
    half & half
    Water

10am

    6oz blueberries
    1/2 cup cooked oatmeal honey
    Water

1pm

    8oz Salmon
    olives endive
    spinach salad
    olive oil vinaigrette
    1/2 hard boiled egg
    Ice tea
    Water
    Ice tea
    Coffee

6pm

    6oz Grilled chicken Cesar salad
    tomato cream sauce
    Water

930pm

    1.5 cup cherries

10pm
Weights
1030pm

    1 tsp peanut butter

Whoa challenging day at work! Crazy busy but loving life and embracing challenges as an opportunity to grow. There is an old saying that may sound cheesy but when the going gets tough, the tough get going! No excuses, be awesome. Don't just show up ...be early! rock the boat! and blow it out of the water. Lets do this!

Day 20

7am
- Water
- Yogurt
- Coffee
- half & half
- Water

1000am
- 4oz blueberries
- cooked oatmeal
- .5 tsp butter
- .5 tsp honey
- Water

120pm
- 1/2 cup tuna
- Tbsp olive oil
- mayo
- celery
- carrot
- 2 cups fresh spinach
- Water

4pm
- nectarine
- 6 almonds
- Water

7pm
- banana
- peanut butter

8pm
yoga
- Water

915pm

yogurt

Today was challenging and it was not just the muffins and fries! Lol I started questioning my new career and whether I am cut out for it, but from what I can tell everyone feels like this at first... its very different, extremely busy, and most of all there is a tremendous amount of pressure to help people find work. Their livelihood depends on me doing my job. It's a huge responsibility but I just have to continue to believe in myself and work really hard and stick to the basics! K.I.S.S.!!!! Most importantly I have to remember God hand placed me there for a reason. And just keep plugging away!!! I felt sore from weights last night and very exhausted after yoga tonight. I can feel the difference in my body and its change and it feels good to be sore and tired because I know its working! !!

Day 21
6am
- Water
- yogurt
- Coffee
- half & half
- Water

9am
- yogurt
- 4oz strawberry
- blueberries
- honey
- Water

1pm
- 2 cups spinach
- 1/2 celery stalk
- 1/2 cup tuna
- olive oil
- mayo
- Water

4pm
- 7 almonds
- Water

7pm
- 2 cups iceberg lettuce
- 1/8 cup ranch dressing

9pm workout
- Water

945pm
- 1 cup nopales cactus
- 2 eggs olive oil

Day 22

7am
- coffee
- half & half

9pm
- 2 blueberry pancakes
- 1 scramble egg
- 1/2 cup home cooked potatoes

1pm
- 1/2 avocado
- turkey sandwich
- wheat bread
- tomato
- alfalfa sprouts
- grapes
- 1/2 large choc chip cookie
- 1 slice carrot cake
- Spaghetti w meat sauce
- 1/2 a garlic toast salad
- ranch
- 2 crackers
- 1/2 pint green tea
- ice cream

Gosh my cheat days are 2 for 2! I always feel like shit had a headache all day used the rest room way too much and felt like vomiting twice. I can tell that my body reacts differently to the sugar in an adverse way. Its like my body is rejecting it. Not sure if the sun or lack of rest had anything to do with it. I'm excited to get back to the program!!!!!

Day 23

8am
- 16oz Water
- 16oz Coffee
- half & half
- yogurt

11am
- 2 oranges
- 8 nuts
- 16oz Water

140pm
- 6oz grilled chicken
- 2 cups mixed spring salad cherry tomatoes
- spicy chipotle dressing
- 16oz Water

420pm
- yogurt
- 5 cherries
- 16oz Water

7pm
- banana
- almond butter

9pm
workout
- 16oz Water

10pm
- broccoli
- peanut butter

I felt much better today getting back to a normal program and just being home. It's been a crazy few weeks so I'm ready to get back into my routine.

Day 24

2am
- banana
- almond butter almond
- milk

7am
- Water
- yogurt
- Coffee
- half & half

10am
- oatmeal
- dried cranberries
- almonds
- honey
- Water

1pm
- 8oz steak sauteed in olive oil 1/2 tomato
- 1/4 avocado spring mix salad
- ranch dressing
- Water

4pm
- 7 almonds
- plum

7pm
- iceberg salad
- cherry tomatoes
- olives
- cucumber
- ranch
- 2 slices Watermelon

9pm weights

930
- nopales cactus
- 2 scramble eggs in olive oil salsa
- Water

12am
- banana w almond butter almond milk
- 2 pinapple chunks

Day 25
7am
- Water
- yogurt

1000am
- strawberry
- blueberries
- yogurt

1pm
- Tuna
- iceberg salad
- 1 plum

4pm
- 2 oranges
- yogurt
- honey

7pm
- yogurt

8pm
yoga

940 pm
- nopales cactus
- scrambled eggs sauteed in olive oil

Was able to twist further in my yoga class today and use my upper body for planks   feeling good feeling leaner.

Day 26
630
- Water
- yogurt
- 16 oz Coffee
- half & half
- Water

930am
- 1/2 cup cooked oatmeal
- honey

        1 Tbsp almond slivers
        dried cranberries
        tsp half and half
        Water

1pm
        2oz chicken sauteed in olive oil
        ranch
        lettuce
        Water

4pm
        6 almonds

7pm
        4oz chicken sauteed in olive oil
        ranch
        Water

8pm
yoga
        Water

915 pm
        yogurt

My first sales day ever and I landed a new account. It's pretty cool to see all my hard work paying off in so many ways. I got a little caught up today and didn't stop myself from working to eat enough. Oh well tomorrow is a new day. Excited to continue to see results and get in some more days at the gym soon. My next goal as I start week 7 and get near to the next phase is to utilize more of the machines at the gym to incorporate more upper and lower body workouts and the trx system.

Day 27
8am
        Water
        yogurt
        Coffee
        half & half

11am
        banana

        peanut butter
        Water

2pm

        6oz steak
        2 cups romaine lettuce
        salsa
        1/2 avocado
        2 Tbsp corn
        vinegrette dressing
        Plain
        ice tea
        lemon
        Water

5pm

        yogurt

730 workout

        Water

9pm

        2 cups steamed green beans 1 tsp butter

1130

        banana peanut butter

Very nice workout today. I felt good having a nice hearty lunch did lots of walking today took my son school clothes shopping. I know I took too long to eat after my workout tonight. I can feel my metabolism speeding up with all the weight lifting. It's so awesome. Looking forward to another great day tomorrow

Day 28

730am

        Water
        Yogurt
        Coffee
        half & half
        Water

1030am

        1/2 cup cooked oatmeal honey
        3 Tbsp almond slivers

dried cranberries
1 tsp half and half
Water

1pm
    1/2 cup tuna with olive oil mayo
    3 cups spring mix
    3 Tbsp balsamic dressing
    Water

3pm
    6 almonds

4pm
    peach
    6 almonds

7pm
    banana peanut butter

9pm
    8 almonds

10pm
    yogurt

1am
    1 cup mixed bluberries raspberries strawberries
    1/2 cup edamame
    1/2 cup fresh orange juice
    1 tsp almond butter
    1/8 cup half & half
    smoothie

I know I should have planned more fiber today tomorrow I will plan my food more carefully. Overall felt great today ... great energy lots of energy. I feel good I feel healthy. I was sore from abs yesterday and my legs were still sore from the deadlifts the day before.

Day 29

7am
    water
    yogurt
    Coffee
    half & half

Water

10am

    1/2 cup cooked oatmeal honey
    1tsp almond slivers
    dried cranberries
    1tsp half & half
    black coffee
    Water

1pm

    6oz roasted chicken
    4oz hummus
    2 cups romaine lettuce
    5 klamato olives
    2 slices cucumber

6pm

    banana
    peanut butter
    Water

8pm
yoga
930pm

    10 oz.steamed peas
    salt
    1 Tbsp butter

1230am

    banana
    frozen peach slices
    1 tsp almond butter
    Water
    2 Tbsp half & half

Whoa sucked again today forgot to eat my snack. I guess I have to set an alarm. Been too busy at work in the afternoon with the meetings. tomorrow I'm Going to have sliced fruit at my desk in front of me. Oh boy i'm feeling hungry before and after work out even while I'm eating. Got to keep fueling the machine and keep this metabolism going! Again went deeper in my twists today in yoga since I don't have all that belly fat in the way. Was able to sink way deeper into my straddle stretch and get my face to the ground.

Day 30
7am
- Water
- yogurt
- Coffee
- half & half

10am
- 1/2 cup cooked oatmeal almonds and dried cranberries
- Water

100pm
- lunch meat
- veggies
- 1 oz cheese
- mayo
- mustard

3pm
- almonds

4pm
- peach almonds

9pm
- yogurt

Weights
10pm
- peanut butter

Ugh another day of planning fail but I made sure to get some extra protein in and my weights. Also lots of water rest and vitamin C!!!

Day 31
8am
- Yogurt
- Water
- Coffee
- half & half

10am
- 1 orange
- Small green apple
- Greek yogurt
- Water

120pm
>2 cups broccoli steamed peanut butter sauce.
>6oz steamed salmon
>red peppers in curry sauce Water

420
>Yogurt
>1 sm apple

720
>Yogurt

945pm
>banana peanut butter

2am
>strawberry
>oranges
>almond butter

Today was sore from weights last night. Yoga was especially challenging I could feel the stretch in my back muscles from last nights weights and we did a lot of leg work. We practiced some dharma yoga. I expect to be sore in my joints knees hips and ankles specifically. What a great workout. I definitely needed that as a balance to my workweek. I think the week work etc. is just catching up to me and I need to make sure I'm getting 8hrs sleep and eating plenty!

Day 32

830am
>Water
>yogurt
>Black coffee

1130am
>Banana
>Peanut butter
>Water

230pm
>6oz chicken
>3 cups iceberg & romaine ranch
>Water

5pm
- 7 almonds
- Water

530
- yogurt

830
- small salad
- ranch
- 1 meatball
- veggie soup
- plain ice tea

Oh wow my triceps and biceps are very sore. I'm so glad I learned some new exercises on the trx! Today was very productive running errands and getting things together for my sons bday. Plus back to school for the kids really excited to move on to the next phase

Day 33

8:40 a.m.
Wake up
- Water

9:20 a.m.
- Yogurt
- Black coffee

11:20 a.m.
- 7 almonds

1145
- 5 strawberries
- Water

230
- 4oz tilapia sauteed in olive oil green peppers
- cantaloupe
- 2 cups spring mix ranch
- Water

Weights

5pm
- banana
- peanut butter

Water
Weights
8pm
    cauliflower & broccoli sauteed in olive oil
1030pm
    yogurt

Today was tough I feel like I'm surrounded by cake and chocolate! Not going to lie I did have a finger full of frosting at one point! Other than that life is good can't complain

Day 34

7am
    Water
    yogurt
    black coffee
    Water

10am
    1/2 cup cooked oatmeal honey
    Water

1pm
    4oz grilled tilapia
    1 slice avocado balsamic dressing
    2 cups spring mix
    Water

4pm
    cauliflower
    carrots
    hummus
    8 almonds

7pm
    yogurt

Abs
10pm
    banana
    peanut butter

Today feeling slimmer and as the days pass I keep craving some fatty foods chocolate and pastries. Lol but when I look in the mirror I remember why I'm working hard and it gets me pumped to keep going. I also think damn when was the last time I had a gassy stomach or felt like shit. And yes it was when I ate like shit! This is what keeps me going I feel great!!!!

Day 35

6am
- Water

630
- yogurt

Weights
- Coffee black
- Water

930
- 1 cup cooked oatmeal
- honey
- Water

1pm
- 6oz chicken grilled
- 3 cups spring mix cherry tomatoes
- 2 tsp grilled sweet corn
- 2 tsp jalapeño jack spicy southwest dressing

4pm
- snow peas
- hummus

7pm
- baked organic squash tomatoes
- 2 Tbsp corn

I have a birthday dinner tonight. Going to eat some high fiber veggies before I go. That is a good feeling when you just continually can pass on birthday cake without batting an eye! I'm so laser focused on my job and NOT hitting a plateau that I will continue to bash and conquer my goals! Relentless! Tiger blood! There is no more mediocre living in the middle for me! Whatever im

doing im not just going thru the motions! I'm absolutely killing it!
Day 36
730
>Water
>yogurt

830
spin class
>Water

1040pm
>yogurt
>Water

120pm
>1 hardboiled egg
>orange
>Water

420pm
>1peach
>peanut butter

700pm
>5 grapes
>2 strawberries

900pm
>8oz fish soup
>carrots
>celery
>tomatos
>onions
>3/4 avocado
>plain ice tea
>Water

Rocked it in spin class! Rode for 40 minutes then called it quits. Didn't want to overdo it! Was able to keep my watts at my body weight and keep my rpm at 80-110. Pretty awesome it felt good to pull my body weight with ease. It's really nice to have people make comments about me looking slimmer. Did well at the baby shower then bbq today. I didn't find any good meat protein at the party so I had tilapia fish soup for dinner. Overate a bit and felt too full. Have not had that feeling in awhile and it did not feel good. But I'm glad I did because it reminded me of why eating smaller portions is important!!!

Day 37

8am

    Water
    yogurt
    Coffee
    1 / 2 cup unsweetened almond milk

11am

    1/2 cup oatmeal
    almond milk
    almonds
    butter
    cinnamon

145pm

    8 oz. chicken
    cabbage
    onion,
    carrots
    broccoli
    lettuce dressing

330pm

    yogurt
    cherries

600pm

    romaine lettuce
    cilantro dressing
    peanuts

Let the fast begin. Definitely felt my diet progress during this yoga class I feel lighter when I'm in plank and chatarunga and less bulky in my obliques when I do a twisted pose. I really feel like I can twist further as my love handles melt away even my boyfriend noticed there is less to hold onto! Lol

I felt good about my last few meals. Drank lots of water and had some herbal tea before bed.

Day 38

Fast all day

    Water
    herbal tea
    black coffee
    1 cup Coffee
    half & half

615pm

    veggie chili
    1/ 2 cup cooked lean ground beef
    1/8 cup crushed tomato
    3 Tbsp corn
    1 cup mushrooms
    1.25 cups squash
    salt & pepper

815
weights
915pm

    1 orange
    greek yogurt
    honey

It felt good to have a nice day to fast I had some errands to run all morning and then to the spa for beatification. It was nice to know that I put the majority of the day into myself. It made me feel so complete and I had some nice reflection time. My thoughts are focused and I'm feeling the rewards of making good choices. I'm also rewarded in my new profession. I would have never imagined my success in life would come from staffing. And yet it's like I found my calling. Helping people find jobs and put food on the table is so fulfilling. My passion and purpose in life is to help people and I know now why God has given me this opportunity: to help others find their purpose and give them the confidence to make good choices. Its like everything makes sense. Overall I had an awesome day. So blessed!

Day 39

2am
>spoonful of peanut butter

730
>Water
>Yogurt
>Coffee
>half & half

1030am
>oatmeal almond slivers dried cranberries
>honey
>Green tea
>Water

1pm
>6oz chicken
>salad romaine spinach iceberg lettuce
>strawberries
>1 tsp sunflower seeds
>1/2 tsp crumbled blue cheese
>apple
>balsamic dressing
>Water

430pm
>nectarine
>peanuts

7pm
>brussel sprouts sauteed in olive oil

10pm
>orange
>yogurt
>honey

Day 40

7am

Water
banana
peanut butter
Coffee
half & half
Water

10am

orange
almonds
Water

1pm

6oz ground chicken
iceberg lettuce salad
chili
lemongrass vinegar cilantro
Water

4pm

peanuts
yogurt
2 orange slices

6pm

peanuts

8pm

yoga
Water

9pm

broccoli
peanut butter
Water

Wow I watched myself doing yoga during my class today. In some poses I almost didn't recognize myself I've really trimmed down in my waist I can see it in my face and neck too. Its great to know I'm making progress. I also know my most stubborn places will go last but I'm not discouraged one bit. I'm excited to keep going and to continue kicking ass at work and in my workouts!

Day 41

7am
- Water
- yogurt
- Coffee
- half & half
- Water

10am
- 6oz blueberries
- 1/2 cup cooked oatmeal honey
- Water

1pm
- 8oz Salmon
- olives endive
- spinach salad
- olive oil vinegrette
- 1/2 hard boiled egg
- Ice tea
- Water
- Ice tea
- Coffee

6pm
- 6oz Grilled chicken
- cesar salad
- tomoto cream sauce
- Water

930pm
- 1.5 cup cherries

10pm
Weights

1030pm
- 1 tsp peanut butter

Whoa challenging day at work! Crazy busy but loving life and embracing challenges as an opportunity to grow. There is an old saying that may sound cheesy but when the going gets tough, the tough get going! No excuses be awesome. Don't just show up ...be early! rock the boat! and blow it out of the water. Lets do this!

Day 42

8am
> Water
> yogurt

11am
> black coffee
> banana

1pm
> 1 cup canteloupe
> Water

5pm
> 8 dorito chips

730pm
> 6oz steak
> 1/2 avocado
> 2 cups romaine
> 1/2 tomato
> 3 Tbsp vinegrette
> water

1030pm
weights

11pm
> yogurt

Ok today again too much going on and I didn't really get to plan my lunch I was so occupied with the party and at some point I had to eat something and yes I had chips which is not like me .. I have not "cheated" at all since I started the program. I don't feel horrible about it but I know it cant happen again. So yes it's all about the preparation!

Day 43

9am
> Water
> yogurt

930
yoga

1130am
> 2 scramble eggs in olive oil salsa
> Black coffee

3pm
- 4oz tilapia sauteed
- olive oil
- 2 cups spring mix
- ranch
- italian dressing
- 1 cucumber
- 1/2 tomato
- Water

5pm
- cherries

8pm
- steamed broccoli
- carrots
- butter

11pm
- yogurt

Another successful day! Feeling good moving forward. I did not do yoga since Tuesday and I could really feel it in my hamstrings and back today when I did yoga. It just lets me see how my body needs yoga 3x a week. I also noticed that I feel better when I do a good weight workout with cardio following twice a week and light weights 2x a week.

Day 44

7am
- Water
- yogurt

8am
- Coffee black

10am
- 1 cup oatmeal
- honey

1pm
- organic squash
- corn
- tomato
- broccoli stew

        1/2 can Tuna w olive oil mayo
        celery stalk
4pm
        7 almonds
7pm
        yogurt
8pm
yoga
10pm
        steamed broccoli
        butter

Overall good day did not feel hungry until about 7pm and then was ready for something light before yoga. Yoga was good I was able to get a good workout and stretch. Starting to feel a bit bloated ... but so far I haven't gained weight so I will just keep pressing on ... yes I'm excited to move and get settled in the new place gonna try and hit a spin class early am before my cheat day!

Day 45
630am
        Water
        yogurt
        black coffee
        Water
11am
        1 cup oatmeal
        honey
145pm
        1/2 can Tuna
        olive oil
        mayo
        iceberg lettuce
        tomato
        shredded carrot
430pm
        7 almonds
730pm
        greek salad

ranch
Water

Lost exactly 2 lbs. Man am I stoked!!! My clothes are getting super loose and I can't wait to continue on with the program and see what the next few weeks will bring. I do feel satisfied with my food. Moving mode all weekend!

Day 46

6am
- Water

645am
- yogurt
- Coffee black
- Water

1030am
- 1 cup oatmeal
- honey
- Water

1pm
- 2 cups ice berg lettuce
- shredded carrots
- red cabbage
- 1000 island dressing
- tomato
- 1 cup bbq beef shredded

4pm
- 4 strawberries
- peanut butter

7pm
- yogurt

8pm
yoga

945pm
- squash
- tomato

Finally back on track. Moving really kicked my butt and I was not able to work out sun or Monday. I was exhausted. I ate well and on track but I missed a few meals and protein here and there. Trying to get back on my grocery list and sleep pattern. It's better today and will be much better tomorrow. Yoga was awesome. It's been a week since i did yoga. My shoulder blades and back were killing me. My back hurts so much from moving it hurts to take deep breaths. I could imagine how I would feel if I didn't work out at all. I would probably be all vicodened out! Overall quality of life is great and happy and fulfilled

Day 47

6am

    Water

630

    yogurt
    Coffee black
    Black coffee
    Water

1030am

    1 cup oatmeal
    honey
    Water

1pm

    6oz grilled chicken
    tomatoes
    2 cups spring mix avocado salsa

4pm

    8 almonds
    2 plums

7pm

    yogurt

830pm

    banana w peanut butter

850
weights

Today was a laborus day. It seemed to take all my will power to get thru it. I was a bad example and bought donuts for the office. I never do that but we had guests and it was hospitable. Better than nothing. I got so many dirty looks when I said I don't eat donuts lol. Anyways trying to finish up the last minute details of the move has taken my energy plus work is draining like treading water all day and moving an inch. But the progress when you reap is worth the hard work. Just gonna keep at it!

Day 48

630am

    Water
    yogurt
    Black coffee

930

    1 cup cooked oatmeal honey
    Water

1230pm

    6oz chicken
    2 cups romaine lettuce carrots
    1000 island dressing
    Water

4pm

    1 tsp peanut butter
    1 peach

7pm

    yogurt

8pm
yoga
10pm

    spinach omelet

Overall good day felt a little hungry right before my yogurt dinner time. But felt really good ay yoga I feel like I can fold my body in half because there is less stomach in the way. Another awesome day!

Day 49

610am

625am
> Water

9am
> yogurt
> Coffee black

1130
> 1 cup cooked oatmeal
> honey
> almond
> Water

1pm
> 7 almonds

330 pm
> 6oz steak
> 2 cups spring mix
> 1000 island
> sunflower seeds

4pm
> almonds

7pm
> peach
> Water

9am
weights
> yogurt
> Water

920
> Water

> peanut butter
> banana

Oh boy really felt slimmer today some of my clothes are so big on me and yes eating is back on track! Felt good today sleep is back on!!! Have to go off site tomorrow. Taking fruit and snacks!!! Oatmeal to go tomorrow am and lots of Black coffee. I hope I get to do yoga tomorrow night!

Day 50

615am
> Water

645
> yogurt
> Black coffee

930
> 1/2 bagel
> cream cheese
> Water
> Black coffee

1230pm
> 4oz ham
> 1 slice swiss cheese
> 1 orange

2pm
> oatmeal cookie

330
> 7 almonds

7pm
> yogurt

Yoga
930pm
> broccoli
> almond butter

Fail to plan. Plan to fail
Training went good then went back to my old apartment to do some final scrubbing for my keys in then went to yoga and I mastered a new pose, which was pretty cool.

Day 51
6am
> Water
> Yogurt
> Coffee black
> Water

9am
> 1 cup cooked oatmeal
> dried fruit
> nuts
> Water

12pm

        1/2 cup tuna
        mayo
        1 slice bread lettuce
        tomato
        1 inch square homemade toffee

3pm
        almonds
        Water

4pm
        1/2 oatmeal cookie
        Water

7pm
        carrot sticks

8pm
        1 tsp almond butter

Ugh another training day and I feel sore still since Sunday so I took a day off

Day 52

630am Water
7am yogurt8am black coffeeWater
10am 1 cup oatmeal with honey
1pm 1/2cup tuna w olive oil mayo Water celery stalk 2 cups spring mix
3pm almonds
4pm strawberries
7pm broccoli steamed with salt and butter.
9pm weights
930pm yogurt

Feeling great physically energy wise. A little stress on the home front had me lacking appetite and forgot to eat here and there over the last few weeks. But I just keep going back to the program!

Day 60

I have lost 16 lbs in 2 months. I feel great and my energy is through the roof. I considered myself healthy before, but I was missing the mark on so many levels. I made all the right adjustments with his encouragement and consulting. I want to thank my food and fitness trainer who is a former professional athlete John Lober. He has changed my whole outlook on life. Not counting what you eat, but eating so your life counts. He has helped with a very deep and emotional transformation for me inside and out.~ Nicole

7. Supplements are the Tune-Ups
A. Liquid Vitamins and mineral.
These are necessary for wellness and longevity. A great company that makes all kinds of this stuff, American Longevity.com. Liquid form, not solid, is the most efficient form of transport in to the blood stream, just like the simple carbs liquify and rush your system.
Couch potato vs. Elite athlete. The couch potato is going to out live the professional elite athlete because they do not sweat as often. When I train, I sweat profusely, and when I do, I am sweating out a soup of essential minerals needed for recovery that I cannot replace through eating just food. They need to be supplemented. Athletes like the famous, Jim Fix and others are dropping dead too early because of cardiovascular disease especially, due to this fact.

B. Vitamin C.
5,000-7,000 IU a day is the only thing that helps prevent or cure the flu virus.

C. Bee Pollen is a complete food and has essential amino acids. Great for the hair and skin also.

D. Creatine
This is the closest you can get to effect of steroids without the side effects. It just be cycled. This supplement makes me tremendously strong, but causes me to retain a lot of water
 in my feet. So, I only use Creatine during recovery, when I have serious injuries, like a shattered shinbone.

E. Steroids/ TRT
Testosterone Replacement Therapy TRT. When an athlete takes a testosterone steroid for any period of time, your nuts recognize this and say, "Hey, were are getting more of this hormone than we need, so

let's shut down and stop producing testosterone." Then the steroid aromatizes and you get cute little bitch titties or you lose your hair and get zits, or all three things happen. And to make it totally awesome, when you run out of testosterone, and your not injecting into your rad body, well your nuts don't turn back on like they forgot how to make it anymore, and you turn into a little bitch. Then you're smart, so you go to the doctor and does a blood test and says your testosterone level is lower than an 80-year old man. So, he writes you a prescription to get back on it as long as you can afford it. You are awesome, but not really at OPL.

F. HGH

Human Growth Hormone is not a hormone or a steroid. It is a chemical that stimulates the pituitary gland in your head to produce the actual hormone. There are a few different brands and it all depends on how many amino acids are in the branch. If you have one that your body is receptive to, then this stuff is amazing for soft tissue healing. You can stay on this as long as you can afford this expensive drug. The Side effects are that it makes the tip of your nose, your jaw and elbows grow excessively if you are on it for an extended period of time. And if you have a tumor that you don't know about, it will triple in size and probably kill you.

G. Natural remedies

Vinegar for heart burn. Heart-burn is causes by a lack of stomached acid, to excess. Like if you drink too much water and dilute the acid, you get heartburn. A swig of Apple cider vinegar causes mucous in the esophagus and lines it and sooths it. Forget the TUMS and Rolaids. Taking Vitamin D for chronically sore feet is a good one also. I also use alcohol and a tiny bit of vinegar to dry and cleanse the ear canal after a shower or swimming.

H. Chiropractic care and Deep tissue Message
When these two are paired together, the results are amazing for speed and strength.

I. Marijuana
Aromatizes to estrogen. That's not good for OPT. But good for Irie mon.

J. Alcohol
Booze creates a catabolic state in your body. That's not Anabolic, and that's not good for OPT, but you're fun at parties, yay!

K. Gakic
This product is designed to remove the waste produced by your muscles immediately for endurance, and it works. Side effects if you take too much you will vomit and your heart may explode. GAKIC is a brand name for a widely available nutritional supplement which, among other ingredients, contains a formulation of the glycine and L-arginine salt of alpha-ketoisocaproic acid calcium. GAKIC is a registered trademark. Clinical studies in humans demonstrate that oral consumption of this formulation enhances muscle performance and recovery from fatigue by sustaining muscle force and work output during intense anaerobic exercise.

L. Meditation and Yoga
I have done all types of Yoga, hot yoga, etc. and I use a sports Hypnosis recording from iTunes from Dr. Rick Collinsworth. The two help relax my mind and strengthen my body. Amazing results.

M. Foam Roller
The black ones are best. If you're waiting for a massage to come, well, it ain't coming, so you better

get acquainted with one of these to roll out muscle soreness and release trigger points in the muscle belly. The roller is great for reducing lactic acid soreness.

N. Melatonin

Melatonin is a hormone found in animals, plants and microbes. I use it mainly to get sound sleep. A minimal dose is required if it is cycled and not abused. I also use Tylenol PM, but not too often because it is hard on my Liver.

8. Testimonial

I've written this recommendation of your work to share with other LinkedIn users.

Details of the Recommendation: "I hired John Lober as a kickboxing instructor in the summer of 2011 and have been extremely satisfied with the results and services offered. After reaching a plateau at a local boxing gym that only offered cardio classes at a basic level I contacted John in order to advance my skills to the next level. I have no aspirations to compete or fight at an amateur level and John has respected this decision and allowed me to work towards my own personal goals of increasing my fitness level while perfecting my skills as a kick boxer.

I have worked with a number of trainers through the years and can say that John is by far my favorite because of the depth of his knowledge and his approach to training. Because of his vast and varied experience as a professional fighter John understands the mechanics of building a skill set. I never feel as though our sessions are haphazard or random – there is always a plan in place and as a result I have seen my fitness level increase greatly and many mechanical issues I had with my kickboxing have been remedied.

John Lober is a man with a high level of integrity who takes his role as a coach in your life very seriously. He is extremely reliable, easy to reach, punctual, and training with him is invaluable. Whether you are a beginner looking for a new training regiment to embark on, or someone like me looking to take your skills beyond the basic level, I give my strongest possible recommendation to John Lober as a trainer." -Susan

Good Luck, Stay Strong and I look forward to hearing from you,

John MACHINE Lober
John Lober's Team Machine
Worldwide/Facebook

Contributing writing credits Nicole Flores

Editing contributor K Keeler www.notjustcalories.com

Made in the USA
Middletown, DE
26 November 2014